PRE-POSTNATAL YOGA WITH ME

ALEXANDRA PAPANIKOLAOU

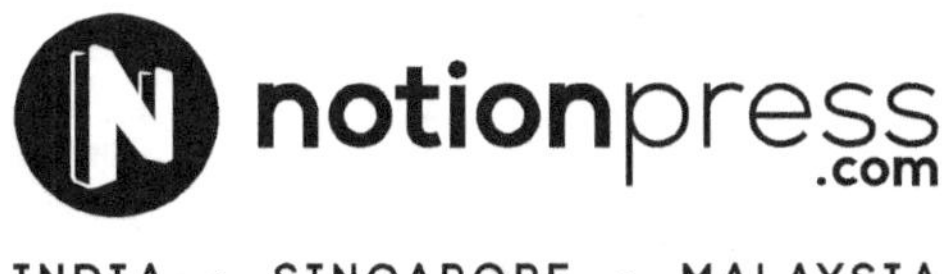

INDIA • SINGAPORE • MALAYSIA

ISBN 979-8-89026-795-5

Dedication

To Nikolas, Philip and Eleana for being my inspiration, motivation and source of prana

Contents

Acknowledgments

During my Reiki Level 1 and 2 training I am grateful I met my Master, Mrs. Taruna Manna, Founder of TARUNAM Holistic, and during my RYT 500HRS I am honored I met my mentor and lead teacher Dr. Anjum Padyal who both have empowered me in so many ways ever since. Amongst many things, they taught me how to be generous with my knowledge gained from my yogic studies. Combining this knowledge with my personal maternal experience, with this book I share the yogic benefits for every woman who wants to explore its gifts, or yoga teachers who seek general information and inspiration on sequencing and cueing.

A special thanks goes to every partner who worked to make this book happen:

- Design Dervish LLP for designing the logo and identity of my brand Yoga With Me.

- The photographers, Bring It Online Media Pvt Ltd and Shivam Bhutani.

- Retreats For Me, which shown me the yogic path with my RYS 200HRS.

- Rishikul Yogshala run under Rishikul Foundation, which gave me all the knowledge and qualification with my RPYS 85HRS Pre-Postnatal Yoga training.

Acknowledgments

- Asht Yoga Institute for Sports and Fitness Development, which helped me find purpose with my studies and also trained me in great detail not only on my RYT 500HRS, but also in Karma Yoga, Yog Nidra, Ayurvedic Nutrition and Therapeutic Yoga.

Nothing of all these would have happened if it was not from the support of my husband, Nikolas.

I am grateful for all the knowledge and experience I gained from all who keep mentoring and supporting my journey.

Introduction

Practicing yoga can only benefit those who choose to yog! Whether you choose to yog to help your body conceive, or you are new to prenatal and postnatal yoga or even experienced and you seek inspiration, in this book you will find guidelines for safe practicing. General information is presented on pregnant body anatomy and physiology, as well as the embryonic development, detailed analysis of asanas per trimester, breathing techniques and mudras. The postnatal period and the first year of motherhood are equally important to conclude the pregnancy journey, as this is the beginning of sharing with the baby the real life experiences and its positive attributes. Yoga, is a wonderful path to share these experiences through co-practicing with the baby asanas, breathing techniques and meditation.

Practicing yoga at these phases of your life can be an amazing journey to find emotional and physical balance and health, with which, one can strengthen and tone up the body, increase prana levels, open up chakra flows, and bring positive changes in life.

With this book I feel the need to pass on to my readers the knowledge and experience I have gained from my pregnancies, endless research in hours and content, studies and qualifications. As a sensible yoga teacher, you should be spending hours researching prenatal yoga before each class! Especially as the pregnancy of your students' progresses, this can be exhausting, since every pregnancy comes with different challenges! The reason for this thoroughness is because baby's health and safety is crucial if giving the would-be-mum inappropriate yoga asanas and breathing exercises. This book is a complete guide for a self-practitioner or a yoga teacher to understand how a pregnancy is developing in order to safely plan pre-postnatal yoga classes per trimester with specific asanas and breathing techniques according to the practitioners' needs, body capacity and mindset.

Disclaimer

Any exercise during pregnancy and during the fourth trimester can pose some level of risk. It is the responsibility of the qualified yoga teacher and any woman who chooses to do yoga to be cautious, practicing by being mindful of safety and fully aware of practitioner's body limits and capabilities. If you are a yoga teacher, it is strongly advisable not to take any risks beyond your guide level of experience, comfort, training and qualifications. If you are a self-practitioner and you have your healthcare advisor's approval to practice Yoga With Me during your pre or postnatal journey, it is advisable to observe your body and whether you experience discomfort or pain, stop the practice at once.

I, Alexandra Papanikolaou, the author of this book take no responsibility for any injury, pain, or other damages caused by the misuse of the content of this book.

Guidelines for Yoga Teachers

One of the most important aspects of a prenatal yoga class is that of fetus' safety, and that of postnatal is safety for the mother and the baby. The teacher's knowledge and skill can guide the students in cautious and effective yoga practicing. It is important to be conservative when teaching prenatal classes, as this is not the time for strenuous practicing or weight loss. Although yoga is a light and gentle form of practice and chances of injuries are low, you need to ensure your insurance is up-to-date and you are fully covered for both yourself and your students.

Ensure your student has medical clearance from her healthcare advisor to practice yoga. If you have concerns, you may also consider signing an indemnity form with your student before start practicing together.

If you are running a yoga studio, it is advisable not to have mixed groups. Women on their first trimester should be having different sequences and cueing from those in second or third trimester. If you decide to take mixed classes, you should be prepared to cue through the class with many modifications and alternative asanas on your sequence, applicable to all trimesters.

Be open to discuss with your students about their expectations attending your classes, as well as their personal experience in pregnancy – both physically and emotionally, so you know in advance how to better sequence your class, but most importantly to urge them to seek advice from their healthcare advisor for matters beyond your capabilities and profession.

When as a teacher you are planning for your yoga classes, consider if your students are new to yoga or experienced. A new practitioner should be practicing mainly poses for beginners, where with your guidance she can connect her body and mind through asanas, breathing techniques and relaxation. An experienced yoga practitioner most probably will know her body capabilities and might be able to describe through own body observation her limitations. Regardless, cautious practicing is the only practicing throughout the four trimesters.

Any jumping or bouncing movement, prone poses, strenuous abdominal exercises, closed or deep twists, deep forward folds and backbends should not be practiced at all during the pre and postnatal duration. From the second trimester onwards should avoid supine positions. A direct supine position to the ground will increase nausea and will also make mobility difficult during practicing. Correct positioning if a supine position is needed, is to use some pillows under the back and spinal cord to bring the upper body to at least 20% inclination. In that way, if we talk about maternal anatomy, the uterus will not compress the inferior vena cava which when compressed can lead to hypotension for the mother, can reduce the blood flow to the baby and in some case can even cause stillbirth.

During pregnancy, balancing asanas should be practiced with safety and caution, better only with the support of a wall, chair or table. The center of gravity changes during pregnancy and a woman can lose her balance a lot easier than before.

Low blood pressure is often experienced during pregnancy, therefore plan your sequence in a way that you always give the counter pose, i.e. rise from a forward bending to standing. A would-be-mum should always move between poses on a slow pace, steadily and mindfully.

All women at this phase of their lives should be encouraged to practice intuitively as they know best what feels right or wrong and at whichever point they might feel discomfort or pain should stop the practice at once. In case discomfort or pain insists and after the practice they should consult their healthcare advisor.

During the fourth trimester and only if there is medical clearance for the practitioner, the Pawanmuktasana Part 2 and 3 may be practiced. The same should be avoided during any phase of the pregnancy due to core engagement and excess pressure in the abdomen area, therefore the womb. With leg raises, the pelvic floor is moving up and down and may have a jerky effect and extra pressure on the belly which can cause more nausea to the woman at this time. In the first trimester it could impact the embryo which is still settling down in the uterus wall (positioned in the pelvic floor) and placenta is not formed yet to protect it. The first trimester is the go-slow-moment when practicing yoga or any other form of exercise. In the second and third trimester, with leg raises, twists and general abdomen activation, extra pressure is forced to the womb and the fragile amniotic sac bag which contains the water called amniotic fluid. Any pressure at this area can harm and suffocate the baby.

Any inverted asanas or asanas with reverse effect can create acidity in the body, because the weight of the baby hits the stomach area, and that is why poses like Ado Mukha Shvanasana or poses where the head is below the heart level are not advisable for practicing. Visualize the left side of the abdomen, where the stomach gets pushed up and squeezed because of the space amniotic sac needs, and below stomach is the spleen, so when baby's weight comes up and hits stomach it results to acidity levels getting aggravated in the body and also can give heart palpitations. As effect of that, woman's blood pressure may also increase.

Make sure there is in place a safety check list of the surroundings, the room temperature should be comfortable, there is easy access to washroom and this is always clean, the fire extinguisher is not expired and fire exits are easily accessible.

First Aid knowledge is advisable. Although it may not be legally required for a yoga studio, it is always good to have such knowledge for your students' reassurance and your personal self-development and confidence to initially handle a possible emergency.

Other than the practical part of running a yoga studio or a yoga class, there is also the theoretical part a good yoga teacher should be very competitive on. The theory of Asanas, Pranayama, Yoga Nidra and Mudras is more important than the practice itself, as through the theory and knowledge gained, you can safely plan an interesting class for your students. You should be having aims and objectives and you should be sharing them with your students on every class. The aims will indicate what your goals are for that particular class, your students will understand better what your expectations and intentions are, and will give you as a teacher a clear path to follow during your class. Objectives will increase your clarity for the class and your targets, as well as your students' capabilities and learning curve.

Unless you are an experienced pre-postnatal yoga teacher, it is always good to consider putting a class plan together, which you have planned with practices to cater both beginner and advanced students, both normal pregnancies and those with various complications. Having a MAP (Modifications, Alternatives and Precautions) can help you cue your class with ease and confidence.

Time consideration will allow you to keep track of your time progress while teaching, which will help on a smoother class experience for you and your students. The classes must always include a 5 to 10 minutes' warm-up, a 5 to 10 minutes' cooling down, in between is the time of asanas' practice where counter poses have to be given, and to finish the class a minimum 5 minutes of relaxation. Breathing techniques are strongly advisable as well as chanting for those who know and feel comfortable with it, are both equally important to the students to help relax the nervous system and bring the body and mind to the present moment of inner peace and tranquility. The duration of pranayama and asanas depends on the booked class duration, and should be planned in precision so each class is complete for maximum students' satisfaction.

Importance of Yoga

Everyone who practices or teaches yoga is aware that every body is not the same and not reacting the same way. Although every body and every person has their own limitations and capacities, yoga's benefits are for everyone, and in particular, practicing yoga for conception, during and after pregnancy will offer women physical, mental, emotional and spiritual benefits.

Thinking of the conception and yoga's importance, it is good to remember that yoga generally creates a positive energy and environment to the practitioner and in this case, a positive environment to welcome the embryo. Promotes physical and mental health and prepares the woman physically, emotionally and spiritually for conception, as yogic practices reduce stress and anxiety. The pranic level and vitality get increased, when at the same time any energy blockages and chakras are opened up. In the physical level, yoga increases body strength, flexibility and endurance of muscles needed for embryo development and later childbirth.

During the prenatal and postnatal period, yoga can benefit a woman Physically, Emotionally and Spiritually and can also benefit the unborn baby.

Physical Benefits

✓ Increases flexibility. With regular practice, flexibility can be increased which will assist with ease of movement, general comfort and well-being throughout a woman's pregnancy journey.

✓ Maintains and Increases Muscle Strength. Everyone who practices yoga regularly with slow and steady movements, can maintain and even increase their muscle strength. During the pre and postnatal journey is particularly important to have muscle strength in order to improve body posture or to help to correct any postural defects that come from pregnancy, i.e. excessive curvature of the lower back. Strengthen the spine and muscles of the back which are under a lot of pressure during pregnancy, as well as the abdominal muscles which support the uterus and baby for 40 weeks and can help on labor process. With muscles' strength, backache can be alleviated and overall health of the physical body can be boosted.

✓ Stronger Pelvic Floor. A pregnant woman's pelvic floor muscles are under a lot of pressure especially during her third trimester and with specific prenatal postures – such as hip opening ones, she can strengthen her pelvic region, create more space in that area and reduce stress put on the abdominal organs. Uterus becomes heavier as pregnancy is progressing, a lot of pressure is put on pelvic floor muscles which loosen up due to body hormonal changes, along with the baby growing, extra pressure is put on the bladder and that can cause urinary incontinence, which is prevented if these muscles are strong. Flexibility of these muscles is beneficial during labor and can prevent tearing. Overall, the physical body is helped and prepared for a natural labor and childbirth.

✓ Increases energy levels. The yogic mindfulness and meditative aspects can help to lower levels of stress and anxiety, which in return will help the woman to feel and be more energetic.

✓ Control over Respiratory System. Helps to gain more control of respiratory system which is needed during labor. With specific chest opening asanas can create more space to make breathing easier, especially in the third trimester when the uterus can press strongly the inner abdominal organs. With asanas and breathing practices can increase oxygen levels for both mother and baby during the pregnancy.

✓ Circulatory and Cardio-Muscular System. During pregnancy, some women experience high or low blood pressure. Through yoga practices, blood cells get oxygenated with proper inhalation/ exhalation, therefore blood pressure can be helped to get balanced and regulated and blood circulation gets improved which in turn strengthens the heart. With proper blood circulation, leg cramps, varicose veins and fluid retention can be prevented and relieved.

Mental, Emotional and Spiritual Benefits

✓ Bond and connection between mother and child. By taking some quite time out when a woman is turning her awareness within, she can tune into deeper connection with baby.

✓ Increases relaxation. When yoga is performed mindfully can help to increase feelings of relaxation, inner peace, concentration and mental clarity. By taking slow, deep breaths, moving mind to a meditative state or even by mentally counting her asanas, a woman can help herself increase mental peace, awareness, calmness, overcome fears, anxiety, conflicts, tension, stress and insomnia which all promote to stress management, leading to emotional wellbeing.

✓ Relieves Anxiety. Prenatal and Postnatal anxiety can be caused by hormonal changes, by body changes, by worries in regards to baby's health, by uncertainty of labor or childbirth or motherhood. Practicing yoga can help balance and stabilize the motions which can be unstable due to hormones and provide some peacefulness and calmness where mum's nervous system can be put at rest and quiet the mind from all thought process.

✓ Awakens Intuition. Through yoga a woman during her pregnancy or postnatal period can calm her mind, thoughts, feelings, opinions, emotions, memories, misconceptions and draw her away from her busy external environment. She can reconnect with her inner wisdom which will allow her to experience positive feelings of love, compassion, appreciation, gratitude, peace, trust and faith in her own body for a more empowered pregnancy and childbirth.

For the Baby

✓ Creates positive energies and a more peaceful atmosphere

✓ Helps in the spiritual development of the baby

✓ Improves blood circulation, removal of metabolic wastes and increased nutrition to the baby

✓ Increases feelings such as care and security for the baby

✓ Promotes a peaceful delivery for the baby

Preparing for Conception

To enter the wonderful journey of pregnancy the couple needs to prepare themselves mentally and physically. If you are planning to become parents, you need to visit the Gynecologist-Obstetrician you feel comfortable with to consult for a personalized advice according to own lifestyle and needs. If you are planning for a pregnancy, the following guidelines are advisable to be taken under consideration, at least 3 months prior to conceiving.

What every healthcare advisor will discuss with you is your personal health history, as well as your family health history. This is important not only for your doctor to know how to consult you throughout your pregnancy, but also seek if needed for further blood tests and examinations. During that first visit, you will need to inform your healthcare advisor of any supplements or medicines you are currently taking, so you can be advised of their safety for the fetus to come; the consultation may result either on change of medication or even stop taking them, as these may harm a pregnancy and the unborn baby. Examples of such medications are usually antibiotics that can cause to fetus amongst others, blood disorders, heart diseases, affect brain development, can even cause miscarriage. Usually, your healthcare advisor at this visit will prescribe for you Folic Acid.

This is the time to start preparing yourselves not only physically, but also mentally, adopt a healthy lifestyle, overcome any fears or barriers you may have, purify yourselves as much as possible. If the one, or both partners are adopting a lifestyle which involves smoking, alcohol consumption, unbalanced diet, or even drugs, these need to be stopped at once, not only for the safe fetus development and having a healthy baby after 40 weeks, but also for personal health benefits. Such habits, especially for the Mother-to-be can make it harder to get pregnant, can cause miscarriage or cause development and health issues to the fetus and later newborn. If you need help quitting these habits, talk to your healthcare advisor.

Regular exercise and discipline on yogic aspects is really important on pre-conception phase and this is because:

- Asanas will prepare the body physically

- Pranayama will give vitality and energy

- Mantras will give prana and mental cleanses

- Yoga Nidra and Meditation in general will help you to overcome possible fears and obstacles

A Balanced Diet is always beneficial for everyone, and since you are preparing for conception, this is the best time to adopt healthy habits, if you are not already doing so:

Reduce		Choose	
✗	Empty calories (ready-made snacks and meals) that contain high processed protein	✓	Eat meals that contain protein, calcium, fiber and whole grain carbohydrates. These good substitutes will help stomach feel fuller for longer durations
✗	Cakes, candies, cookies	✓	Eat fresh, local, seasonal fruits and vegetables, grains and dairy products
✗	Artificial sweeteners	✓	Use jiggery or coconut sugar
✗	Branded cereals contain too much sugar	✓	Start eating plain oatmeal
✗	Caffeine intake (maximum 2 cups a day)	✓	Drink plenty of water or herbal tea
✗	Sitting for too long	✓	Exercise

For a woman who is regularly exercising before conceiving, her body can deal a lot easier with the changes pregnancy and labor will give to her mind and body. It is safe to exercise during pregnancy, however, each pregnancy is unique, and no matter how fit or confident a woman feels, should always consult healthcare advisor and discuss preferred type of exercise, ideal duration and frequency.

On the other hand, if a woman is not regularly exercising, during the pre-conception period it is advisable to start at least a 30 minutes of Brisk Walk 4 to 5 times a week on the nearest park, the beach, the hills, the city, wherever you find ease, joy and comfort doing so. Yoga is widely accepted for everyone from 5 to 100 years old, as such, during conception phase can help the couple to control their sexual energy and with particular series of asanas the reproductive organs can also be benefited.

The same list of asanas given for Pre-Conception can also be practiced during the Postnatal recovery phase. During this time, a woman may be already carrying and not be aware of that as yet, therefore, cautious practicing is always advisable. From the moment she senses she may be pregnant and not yet have it confirmed, it is again advisable to practice gentle asanas and follow the First Trimester guidelines. Until that moment, pre-conception is a time when all asanas can be practiced according to personal physic and body capacity, however, more focus should be given as a combination to Pawanmuktasana Part 1, Relaxation, Meditation and Vajrasana Group of Asanas to help the willing pregnancy to be.

Anatomy and Physiology

As a prenatal yoga teacher or as a self-practitioner, you need to understand the pregnant woman's anatomy in order to plan safe and effective classes. It is important to have at least basic knowledge in maternal anatomy in order to have a better understanding of how a woman's body is changing throughout pregnancy, what she may be experiencing and how she might be feeling physically and emotionally so you can design yoga classes that can help her in that journey.

It is important to remember, we as yoga teachers are not doctors (unless you hold such qualifications). We have to work with a sensitive body – physically and emotionally, and every body is different, as every pregnancy is. Our knowledge comes from studying and practicing yoga and although our human anatomy studies can give us a clear understanding of how body functions, it is advisable not to give suggestions to your students nor medical advice. Always refer them to their healthcare advisor for questions or worries about their body and unborn baby. We are here to help a woman during her pregnancy and the first year of her motherhood for her to feel calm, relaxed, rejuvenated and achieve her goals, whether these are about her body, mind, health or wellness.

Pregnancy is the time from conception to birth and occurs after egg and sperm are combined (fertilization) and the fertilized egg becomes a zygote. The zygote then undergoes cleavage (mitosis) for 6-10 days when it attaches to the uterus and develops into an embryo which further grows to a baby.

Getting pregnant and being pregnant is a very complicated biological process that takes a lot of resources and medical studies. What is known is that pregnancy can effect a woman both physically and emotionally.

Herein, it will be analyzed the basics someone needs to know for own pregnancy or how to safely guide a Pre and Postnatal Yoga Class.

During the menstrual cycle, each released egg travel to uterus. The unfertilized eggs travel unaltered and when they reach uterus get disintegrated. A fertilized egg, while traveling to uterus through the fallopian tube, develops into a tiny human embryo. As soon as the embryo reaches the uterus, implants itself in the uterine wall and the woman is now called pregnant, whereas the embryo develops into a fetus which steadily grows until it is ready for birth.

For a woman being fertile and sexually active, the first thing she is likely to notice is a missing menstrual period (amenorrhea) when she becomes pregnant. The process of fertilization initiates hormonal changes almost immediately, that continue through the pregnancy to help the growth of a healthy baby. These changes can cause swollen breasts, fatigue, dizziness, nausea and vomiting.

Hormones

Each pregnancy and post-pregnancy is implicitly connected to the endocrine system. As yoga teachers, we don't need to know the endocrine system in detail, all we need to know is some key hormones secreted during pregnancy and that hormones are the body's chemical messengers secreted directly into the bloodstream traveling to organs and tissues which affect body functions and processes, such as growth, development, metabolism, cognitive function. In pre conception phase hormones can affect sexual function and reproductive health. During pregnancy, hormone levels change dramatically to assist baby's development. A number of hormones are secreted from the moment of fertilization until childbirth and during breastfeeding.

Relaxin

Relaxin hormone loosens up the ligaments and skeletal muscles that hold the pelvic bones together and also the cervix to ease labor. This loosening, particularly in the first trimester when relaxin levels are highest, needs to be taken seriously as the woman needs to adjust her yoga asanas and be careful not to overstretch.

Walking is generally advised by many doctors and obstetricians for a healthy pregnancy as this is a light exercise with important benefits to human systems. Yoga is also a very helpful way of exercise to trigger and relax the mind from stress, and help the changing body to keep its fitness, flexibility and balance.

HCG

Human Chorionic Gonadotropin (HCG), cannot affect in any way the yoga practice, however it is important to be mentioned as this is the key hormone during a pregnancy. HCG works as a protective shield for the baby and can be detected in the maternal urine approximately 8 to 10 days after fertilization. Its principal function is to let the woman's body know there is a growing life inside her womb until the placenta is sufficiently developed to take over production of progesterone.

Progesterone

With fertilization, progesterone hormone is secreted to prepare uterus for the implantation of a fertilized egg – the pregnancy, until the placenta takes over. Progesterone increases the blood flow to the womb which is important for the healthy development of the fetus, however, this might be a cause for heartburns, morning sickness, reflux, gas and constipation. Can also relax the blood vessels effecting to lower blood pressure which can cause dizziness during pregnancy. As the pregnancy progresses, prevents lactation until baby is born with the growth of maternal breast tissue and strengthens pelvic floor muscles for labor.

Estrogen

During the beginning of pregnancy, estrogen is produced for placentas' correct functioning and for baby's organs' development. The production of estrogen may cause nausea, and relaxation of ligaments and joints in the body which leads to extra pressure on lower back and pelvis area. From second trimester, the increase of estrogen levels prepares the body for lactation and breastfeeding that causes breasts' enlargement, tenderness and/or swollenness; also enables uterus to respond to oxytocin during labor.

Oxytocin & Prolactin

Oxytocin is produced in the hypothalamus and is secreted to the bloodstream. During the third trimester, stimulates contraction of uterus and encourages cervix to open and ease labor. After labor, oxytocin and prolactin hormones are both responsible to activate the mammary glands for milk production, the so called lactogenesis. Both oxytocin and prolactin hormones can trigger increased secretion with breastfeeding and while mother-baby hugging, kissing, cuddling can further help on their bonding.

With all the hormonal and physiological changes in a woman's body during her pregnancy, it is very common to experience fatigue, as well as be emotionally down or anxious at times. Experiencing such feelings during pregnancy may lead to postnatal depression, so it is advisable to encourage your students to talk about their pregnancy experiences and may you direct them to their healthcare advisor or someone close to them in case you identify issues beyond your ability and knowledge to handle.

Common Conditions during Pregnancy

Herein this chapter is presented in short the most common pregnancy experiences a woman may have during this journey and how yoga can assist to ease these conditions. Always, as a yoga teacher you should refer your student back to her healthcare advisor for medical advice, however, in this book you will get the asanas you should and should not practice according to the condition.

Back Pain

Back pain is maybe one of the most common condition during a pregnancy. The weight the woman is carrying from the weight she has put on, as well as the growing weight of her baby can put extra pressure on her muscles, connective tissue and joints.

If she generally experiences back pain, she should avoid any strong asanas, should practice with caution, use props such as cushions if needed. Especially with forward bends she should keep her feet parallel, putting awareness on the posture, avoid standing on one leg more than the other, as well as avoid lying on her back for long durations.

Yoga gentle stretches can release some of the back pain. Also, with prenatal yoga the muscles of the back and the core, including the pelvic floor muscles can be strengthened. Some of the asanas you may consider for back pain:

- Bridge or Shoulder Pose – Kandharasana or Setu Bandha Sarvangasana

- Camel Pose – Ushtrasana

- Cat and Cow Stretch Pose – Marjariasana

- Half Camel Pose – Ardha Ushtrasana

- Half Forward Bend – Ardha Uttanasana

- Seated Camel Pose – Ushtrasana in Sukhasana

- Seated Spinal Twist – Parivritti in Sukhasana

- Standing Spinal Twist Pose – Katichakrasana

Pelvic Girdle Pain

Pelvic Girdle Pain (PGP) or Symphysis Pubis Dysfunction (SPD) affects 1 in 5 pregnant women and is caused by misalignment or stiffness of the pelvic joints. PGP cannot harm the unborn baby, but can be painful for the would-be-mum over the front of the pubic bone, over one or both sides of the lower back, pain in the perineum area, which pain can be spread to the lower back, groin and thighs. 1

If a woman has severe pelvic or abdomen pain in the first trimester it can indicate a tubal pregnancy, when in the third trimester it could be a placental abruption. Both cases are considered emergencies and no asana practice should be taken. She should contact her healthcare advisor at once for pain management or treatment.

When suffering from PGP, one should avoid practicing for too long any standing asanas, especially standing on one leg, bending or twisting, sitting on the floor, especially with crossed legs. Avoid opened legged asanas, but if still practicing the would-be-mum should find her own pain-free angle and not force any asana what-so-ever.

With the following asanas she can strengthen the spine, pelvic floor, stomach, back and hip muscles.

- Bird Dog or Balancing Table Top Pose – Parsva Balasana

- Bridge or Shoulder Pose – Kandharasana or Setu Bandha Sarvangasana

- Cat and Cow Stretch Pose – Marjariasana

- Extended Puppy Pose – Uttana Shishosana

- Gate Pose – Parighasana

Hernia

A hernia is when an internal organ or a fatty tissue pushes through a weakened area in the abdominal muscles or tissue wall. It can be developed anywhere between the chest and hips area; it usually has no or only a few symptoms such as swelling or lump. During pregnancy we are mostly concerned with the abdominal hernias which can occur as the pregnancy progresses and the developing fetus can add extra abdominal pressure.

It can be diagnosed with an ultrasound and the mum-to-be will need to visit her healthcare advisor to discuss treatment option for her hernia.

No asana that will put pressure to the abdomen should be practiced during pregnancy, and especially if the woman is suffering from hernia. Any asana that takes pressure away from the abdomen area can be practiced.

- Camel Pose – Ushtrasana

- Extended Puppy Pose – Uttana Shishosana

- Full Butterfly – Poorna Titali Asana

- Legs Up The Wall Pose – Viparita Karani

- Sleeping Thunderbolt Pose – Supta Vajrasana

- Thunderbolt Pose – Vajrasana/ Virasana

- Triangle Pose – Trikonasana

Diastasis Recti

The growing uterus is putting extra pressure to the abdomen area and pushes the muscles apart, making them longer and weaker. It is common during a pregnancy to have these muscles pulled apart, especially when the abdomen muscles are weak, either due to lack of exercise, or multiple pregnancies, or over exerting. The abdomen area muscles' separation usually returns to normal by the 8th or 10th week post childbirth.

If a woman has diastasis recti she should consult her healthcare advisor on the condition. She should not practice any asanas that strain or stretch the abdominal muscles, such as backbends, side bends and twists. It is safe to practice Kegel exercises and side stretches.

- Extended Side Angle Pose – Utthita Parsvakonasana

- Seated Side Bend – Parsva Sukhasana

- Standing Pelvic Rotation

- Swaying Palm Tree Pose – Tiryak Tadasana

Incompetent Cervix

Incompetent Cervix is when the cervix during the pregnancy has softened too early and may begin to open earlier than normal causing premature labor. The would-be-mum most probably has been advised by her healthcare advisor to bedrest and limit her activity and exercise.

• Pawanmuktasana Part 1

• Seated Eagle Pose – Garudasana

• Seated Side Bend – Parsva Sukhasana

Piles

Piles or Hemorrhoids are common during pregnancy due to excess pressure on the abdomen, constipation and weakening of the pelvic floor muscles.

Avoid full Squatting Asanas such as Kaliasana, as these will aggravate the condition. Instead, asanas to tone up the pelvic floor muscles are most advisable.

• Cat and Cow Stretch Pose – Marjariasana

• Dog Pose – Shvanasana

• Full Butterfly – Poorna Titali Asana

• Half Forward Bend – Ardha Uttanasana

• Thunderbolt Pose – Vajrasana/ Virasana

• Warrior II – Virabhadrasana II

Low Blood Pressure

Low blood pressure and faintness is common during pregnancy due to the increased demand for blood for both the mother and the growing fetus. The increased progesterone which relaxes the blood vessels' wall may also be the reason for low blood pressure and faintness.

It is safe to practice yoga with this condition, as long as the practice movements are slow with extra care when changing positions, i.e. from forward fold up to standing poses, avoid standing or practicing on supine positions for too long. When following the slow movements or half way movements, the woman allows her blood pressure to normalize. Any asana which positions the head below the heart may cause dizziness, nausea or faintness.

If the would-be-mum feels faint during the practice, ask her to lie down on the side until she feels better and discontinue the practice for the day.

- Child's Pose – Shashankasana

- Extended Side Angle Pose – Utthita Parsvakonasana

- Flapping Fish Pose – Matsya Kridasana

- Triangle Pose – Trikonasana

- Warrior I – Virabhadrasana I

High Blood Pressure

High blood pressure is common during pregnancy and should be treated seriously, as in some cases it can signal a condition called pre-eclampsia. Students with pre-eclampsia should be under medical supervision and should be limiting their exercise according to doctor's consultation.

Brisk walking, swimming and yoga are considered safe forms of exercise for those with high blood pressure. When practicing yoga, any inverted asanas, standing forward bends and poses that feel uncomfortable should not be practiced at all. Safe yoga practicing includes asanas where the head is above the heart level:

- Duck Walking – Karandavasana

- Legs Up The Wall Pose – Viparita Karani

- Reclined Butterfly Pose – Supta Baddhakonasana

- Seated Camel Pose – Ushtrasana in Sukhasana

- Seated Spinal Twist – Parivritti in Sukhasana

- Warrior I – Virabhadrasana I

- Warrior II – Virabhadrasana II

Gestational Diabetes

Gestational Diabetes will be diagnosed for the first time during a pregnancy and usually will disappear after childbirth. It can cause If it is elevated in early pregnancy it may be possible to cause certain birth defects or even miscarriage at rare cases. If it is elevated in the advance stages of pregnancy, it could cause respiratory distress in the growing fetus and is also linked to prolonged labor.

A would-be-mum can continue to practice asanas and pranayama and should include on the classes relaxation time. Such students should always have the clearance from their healthcare advisor. As a yoga teacher, you must always advise the would-be-mum prior to a class to monitor and observe how she feels during practice and should take more breaks with breathing techniques.

- Child's Pose – Shashankasana

- Corpse Pose – Shavasana

- Head to Knee Pose – Janu Sirshasana

- Seated Palm Tree Pose – Parvatasana in Sukhasana

- Seated Side Bend – Parsva Sukhasana

- Seated Spinal Twist – Parivritti in Sukhasana

- Side-Reclining Leg Lift Pose – Anantasana

Oedema, Swelling or Varicose Veins

Oedema or swelling in the fingers and lower limb, especially in the ankles and the forefoot, is common in most pregnancies. It can be caused by excess fluid in the tissues and also by the extra blood produced to help fetus healthy development. The uterus can press and affect the blood flow in the lower limbs and can cause pooled fluid particularly in the legs, ankles and feet, which can produce swelling. A sudden swelling may be a sign of pre-eclampsia, in which case it is strongly advisable for the would-be-mum to see her healthcare advisor immediately.

With yoga, blood circulation can be boosted and can also reduce swelling and varicose veins. One should avoid standing for too long, always wear comfortable shoes, drink plenty of water, rest feet up as often as possible, practice foot stretches.

- Ankle Bending – Goolf Naman

- Ankle Rotation – Goolf Chakra

- Extended Supine Hand to Big Toe Pose – Utthita Supta Padangusthasana

- Full Butterfly – Poorna Titali Asana

- Half Butterfly – Ardha Titali

- Legs Up The Wall Pose – Viparita Karani

Carpal Tunnel Syndrome

Carpal Tunnel Syndrome (CTS) occurs when the wrists' nerves receive pressure. It can cause tingling, numbness, and aching in the forearm, hands, wrist and fingers.

Generally, avoid any asanas that will put weight on the wrists, such as tabletop postures. If you are about to practice a tabletop asana, it is advisable to modify it onto the forearms or on standing.

Practice the elbow, hand, shoulder and wrist asanas from the Pawanmuktasana Part 1.

Leg Cramps

Leg cramps are mostly experienced during late pregnancy and are sudden pains in the calf muscles, feet or thighs. Usually these are experienced during the sleep and can be uncomfortable and painful.

Calf muscles stretches are helpful in leg cramps and it is advisable to practice them at bed before sleeping at night.

- Ankle Bending – Goolf Naman

- Ankle Rotation – Goolf Chakra

- Bird Dog or Balancing Table Top Pose – Parsva Balasana

- Half Forward Bend – Ardha Uttanasana

- Side-Reclining Leg Lift Pose – Anantasana

- Wide Angled Seated Forward Bend – Upavistha Konasana

Sciatic Pain

Sciatic pain occurs when the sciatic nerve which runs from lower back through the hips and buttocks and down to each leg is irritated or compressed. In pregnancy, the sciatic nerve runs below the uterus and it can be irritated or compressed by the weight of the growing fetus. It is usually felt only on one side of the body, however, if felt on both sides, should contact healthcare advisor immediately and may be required to have physiotherapy.

Avoid supine postures, any strong asanas, standing on one leg more than the other and for long durations, extending too far on forward folds. Instead, should be gentle with all practices, use of cushions if needed – especially with forward bends and should be placing extra awareness in the posture of each asana. Gentle back stretches, extensions or twists may release some of the weight of the nerve. However, because there are different causes of sciatica, some asanas may aggravate the condition, therefore she needs to move gently, slowly and mindfully when practicing.

If at any occasion she feels pain while practicing yoga, she should come out of these poses.

- Base Position – Prarambhik Sthiti

- Bridge or Shoulder Pose – Kandharasana or Setu Bandha Sarvangasana

- Extended Side Angle Pose – Utthita Parsvakonasana

- Goddess Pose – Kaliasana

- Half Forward Bend – Ardha Uttanasana

- One-Legged King Pigeon Pose – Eka Pada Rajakapotasana

- Salutation Pose – Namaskarsana

- Side-Reclining Leg Lift Pose – Anantasana

- Warrior I – Virabhadrasana I

Inferior Vena Cava Syndrome

During pregnancy and especially from second trimester onwards, when a would-be-mum is on supine position, the uterus compresses the inferior vena cava which in turn reduces dramatically the blood flow in the inferior vena cava. This can cause dizziness while on supine positions or when laying on right side.

During yoga practices, it is strongly recommended to always instruct your students to come up from a supine position from left side to avoid being lightheaded of dizzy, or could be positioned in an inclined position with the use of a bolster or cushions.

- Flapping Fish Pose – Matsya Kridasana

- Reclined Butterfly Pose – Supta Baddhakonasana

- Seated Cat & Cow Pose – Marjariasana

- Seated Palm Tree Pose – Parvatasana in Sukhasana

- Seated Prayer Flow – Sukhasana Namaste Hands Vinyasa

- Side-Reclining Leg Lift Pose – Anantasana

Weight Gain

Pregnancy is a 40-weeks journey of constant and non-stop internal developments to support a healthy support system for baby's growth and woman's ability to keep up with her own demands. At this time, it is normal to gain some weight due to baby's growing weight, placenta and amniotic fluid. Women or people around them tend to believe that during her pregnancy a woman should be eating for two! That is not true, and it only depends on pre-pregnancy Body Mass Index (BMI). The healthcare advisor can help on accurate BMI calculation and can either help monitor the weight or can refer mother-to-be to a specialized nutritionist.

Components to consider for the extra weight is how much each component weights during the pregnancy and at childbirth. On average, the following table shows the weight of the fluids that will be lost after childbirth, the storing of nutrients that lead to actual extra weight and the baby's weight at childbirth.

Component Parts	Weight
Amniotic Fluid	0.9 kg
Placenta	0.7 kg
Growth of Uterus	0.9 kg
Growth of Breasts	1.1 kg
Increased Amount of Blood	1.5 kg
Increased Amount of other Body Fluids	1.1 kg
Storing of Nutrients (fat and protein)	3.1 kg
Baby's Weight	≈ 3.0 kg
Total Weight	**12.3 kg**

Malnutrition can lead to weight loss for the would-be-mum's body, and not enough and healthy eating can lead to not gaining enough weight during pregnancy, which may increase the chances of a preterm childbirth or a smaller baby born.

On the other hand, excess weight gain during a pregnancy can increase chances of high blood pressure and/or gestational diabetes. May also increase chances having a larger baby for birth which might need a caesarean section and later for baby's life can increase the risk of obesity. Thinking of the postnatal body, excess weight gains in pregnancy due to eating habits will create a difficulty to weigh loss or even weight management.

- Airplane Pose – Kati Sakti Vikasaka

- Dog Pose – Shvanasana

- Donkey Kicks Straight Raised Leg

- Duck Walking – Karandavasana

- Goddess Pose – Kaliasana

- Half Forward Bend – Ardha Uttanasana

- Lizard Pose – Utthan Pristhasana

- One-Legged King Pigeon Pose – Eka Pada Rajakapotasana

- Side-Reclining Leg Lift Pose – Anantasana

- Spiraled Head to Knee Pose – Parivritti Janu Sirshasana

- Triangle Pose – Trikonasana

- Warrior I – Virabhadrasana I

- Warrior II – Virabhadrasana II

Emotional Issues

It is common during a pregnancy a woman to experience psychological swings. During that journey, a flood of massive pregnancy hormones occurs that make every emotion to be felt more intensely, where a woman can start crying or getting angry for no particular reason or over-exaggerate about minor things.

The change on emotions affect her relationships, particularly the one with her partner. It can be difficult for him to understand or feel what the woman may be going through – physically and emotionally, however, his role takes a serious part during the pregnancy, as he also needs to change along the pregnancy journey and also offer to his partner all the love, reassurance, intimacy and care she needs, for her to feel supported and secure. It can also be a challenging period for the mother-to-be, as emotional changes are happening to him as well, since the relationship no longer involves just them two, and responsibilities and worries and fears may rule his mind too.

These psychological issues can be caused by stress about the unborn baby, her relationship with mother-to-be or family issues, financial issues, prior mental health problems. If we talk about symptoms of that emotional state in the physical body, these could be insomnia, high blood pressure, muscle tension, neck and shoulder pain, fatigue, heartburn. Psychological and emotional symptoms could be anxiety, nervousness, irritability, crying, unbalanced nutrition, lack of concentration.

Along with counseling, it is important for the partners to communicate their thoughts and worries and love and care for each other. Yoga can help both to be better physically and emotionally and they should focus on asanas, pranayama, mantra chanting if they are familiar, visualization techniques when practicing Yoga Nidra and meditation, but most important, practice gratitude for the gift of life.

- Camel Pose – Ushtrasana

- Cat and Cow Stretch Pose – Marjariasana

- Chair Pose – Utkatasana

- Child's Pose – Shashankasana

- Easy Pose – Sukhasana

- Extended Puppy Pose – Uttana Shishosana

- Half Camel Pose – Ardha Ushtrasana

- One-Legged Prayer or Tree Pose – Eka Pada Pranamasana

- Swaying Palm Tree Pose – Tiryak Tadasana

- Warrior I – Virabhadrasana I

The Pregnant Body – First Trimester

The body of a woman during pregnancy changes externally and internally. As she progresses on her pregnancy, the digestive organs will adjust to accommodate the baby. Usually, a pregnancy lasts up to 40 weeks or 280 days, generally referring to 9 months and its progress is divided into three trimesters.

The timeframe for the first trimester is between 1-12 weeks of pregnancy and can be called the embryogenesis.

During the first trimester, although not much can be observed on the outer body, the inner body is working rigorously to develop a healthy environment and a life-supporting system for the embryo. The secretion of hormones builds up the uterine lining, and the increase in blood volume facilitates this construction. It is common to have lower blood pressure than usually had, because the heart needs this drop to be able to pump extra blood to support baby's growth. Muscle tissue begins to relax, particularly in the abdomen area, and joins start to loosen up so the uterus is allowed to stretch during the whole pregnancy to create a healthy home environment for the baby-to-come.

During the whole pregnancy, the first 10-12 weeks are the most critical and with the highest risk for miscarriage. It is advisable to limit physical activity or practice yoga in a light form, as we need to insure implantation of embryo in the uterus and also placenta's proper attachment.

On the physical level, if the mother-to-be is experiencing morning sickness, possibly won't see much change on her weight. However, typically there is an increase in weight of approximately 1 or 2 kg, which occurs from the placenta formation, the enlargement of breasts, the growing uterus and extra blood. Because the body is working to produce more blood to support baby's healthy development, she might feel lightheaded. If she feels fatigue, nausea, faintness or dizziness is common during the first trimester. She may feel her breasts tender, heavier and tingling because of its enlargement. The growth of uterus will start putting more pressure to the bladder which in turn will increase the need to urinate. The slow breakdown of food and oral iron supplements can create bloating, heartburn, indigestion and constipation.

On the mental level, her emotions may become unstable with positive or negative mood swings, which occur due to hormonal changes. Mixed feelings, fear, confidence, readiness, changes to come, may play a key role on her thought process – which overthinking can create some short of stress, which in turn can cause insomnia.

It is important to keep reminding the practitioners they need to practice with awareness on the embryo's safety, while introducing a more introspective yoga practice, where any new, advanced or strenuous practices for the pregnant body should be avoided. If the mother-to-be is an experienced yoga practitioner, she may be able to continue her regular practice with modifications, following healthcare advisor's and pregnancy guidelines. In such case, she will have a good understanding of the yogic principles of comfort, safety, stability and body awareness, where a non-experienced practitioner should always practice in the presence of an experienced and qualified prenatal yoga teacher. In both cases all pregnant women must be encouraged to observe and listen to their body and should not overstretch, strain or push.

This is also the time which the woman may decide to announce her pregnancy or keep it a secret until she reaches the second trimester when her pregnancy is most settled. Many people as soon as they find out about a pregnancy they tend to share positive and negative stories about others' or own pregnancy and childbirth. In any case, it is always best to surround herself only with positivity and plenty of calmness and relaxation both for her own benefits and her growing embryo.

If we talk about yogic practices, during the beginning of a pregnancy, most of basic yoga asanas can be practiced, but always respect practitioners' instinct while practicing and always support self-awareness for what body is feeling and its' own capacity.

During this time, sudden dizziness may be experienced, therefore all Standing and Balance Asanas should be practiced near a wall or with the support of a wall for better balance. Such asanas are all strengthening the leg muscles and the pelvic floor area which needs to be prepared particularly for the third trimester and childbirth. Also, these enhance blood circulation, particularly in the lower limps to prevent cramping, swelling, edema or even varicose veins.

- Chair Pose – Utkatasana

- Extended Side Angle Pose – Utthita Parsvakonasana

- Extended Triangle Pose – Utthita Trikonasana

- Goddess Pose – Kaliasana

- One-Legged Prayer or Tree Pose – Eka Pada Pranamasana

- Triangle Pose – Trikonasana

- Warrior I – Virabhadrasana I

- Warrior II – Virabhadrasana II

- Warrior III – Virabhadrasana III

Any strong twists, standing or seated should be avoided due to the excess pressure on the abdominal area. However, open and closed seated twists alleviate lower back pain and also encourage correct body posture by loosening the vertebrae.

- Airplane Pose – Kati Sakti Vikasaka

- Head to Knee Pose – Janu Sirshasana

- Seated Side Bend – Parsva Sukhasana

- Seated Spinal Twist – Parivritti in Sukhasana

- Spiraled Head to Knee Pose – Parivritti Janu Sirshasana

Hip opener asanas should be at the main focus of every practical session during a pregnancy, as these increase pelvic floor flexibility which is vital for childbirth. Awareness while practicing hip opener asanas should be on gentle stretching and should never over-stretch even if it feels comfortable. Relaxin hormone during pregnancy is softening all the joints and if a practitioner overstretches can dislocate joints.

- Full Butterfly – Poorna Titali Asana

- Wide Angled Seated Forward Bend – Upavistha Konasana

Supine stretches and especially the reclining ones are good as these help on digestive ailments and constipation, work on making the back more flexible and loosen up the leg muscles to also prepare for delivery. It is always important to remember to avoid any overstretching of the abdominal region, as this is a delicate time for the uterus. Cushions, yoga blocks, bolsters or pillows can be used to ease the practices.

- Extended Supine Hand to Big Toe Pose – Utthita Supta Padangusthasana

- Reclined Butterfly Pose – Supta Baddhakonasana

- Sleeping Thunderbolt Pose – Supta Vajrasana

- Universal Spinal Twist – Shava Udarakarshanasana

Inverted poses should be avoided during a pregnancy because we need to avoid blood circulation moving away from the uterus. Also, those who may experience low blood pressure, may have an increased effect of dizziness. However, as an exception to the inverted poses is the Mountain Pose – Parvatasana which can be fine to practice but only for short periods of time, without any pulsing and the would-be-mum should adjust her body positioning to her comfort level.

On any seated poses, legs should be closed on. If need to practice asanas with legs wider open, keep the distance between the legs maximum to the width of the yoga mat. From the yogic point of view, while on First Trimester, we emphasize on sitting with legs closed, as the pelvic floor is governed by Apana Vayu, the Downward Moving Energy, which we aim to maintain at this initial stage of pregnancy. We should not activate this downward moving energy, as it pushes things down in an accelerated mode and there is risk of miscarriage. If we talk scientifically, at this stage embryo is still getting settled and placenta is not fully formed yet – at least not until the end of first trimester, so any type of opening up of the cervix area and birth canal can create jerky effect on the internal parts of the pelvic floor. However, for certain practices a woman can practice differently with her full awareness on the movement so that there is no jerk on the pelvic area.

During the first trimester, the physical body is working in high demand to develop a safe and healthy environment for the fetus, and the energy levels of the mother-to-be usually are low, therefore, high energy sequences, power yoga, Sun or Chandra Salutations, jumping practices and any abdominal muscle stretches should be totally avoided.

Pranayama can be extremely helpful, relaxing and energetic at the same time, for both mother-to-be and also the embryo that still develops its own prana source up until the end of first trimester. Pranayama techniques have also a strong effect to the mind and mindset and can help increase focus and concentration, reduce stress and anxiety and also control the unbalanced emotions due to hormonal changes.

Relaxation with inclined modified Shavasana or Matsya Kridasana, Yoga Nidra, Visualization or Meditation are very much important practices to calm the body and mind. Yoga Nidra will help increase energy levels, whereas visualization and meditation can prepare the mental and body state for the pregnancy, childbirth and newborn; all practices with main goal a positive aspect for the mother-to-be and the baby.

The Pregnant Body – Second Trimester

The timeframe for second trimester is between 13-28 weeks of pregnancy, when by the fifth month pregnancy usually becomes visible. Every woman and every pregnancy is different, although some women feel more energetic and find this trimester easier than the first one, in terms of morning sickness, nausea and fatigue that usually settle down by second trimester. However, some may have these symptoms throughout the whole pregnancy. It is this trimester when the mother-to-be may begin to feel baby movements, and that usually happens around 18-22 weeks.

The abdomen is expanding as baby grows and the breasts become larger and fuller as the apparatus develops for nursing. The mother-to-be may develop darker skin patches in the cheeks, forehead, nose and/or upper lip, which sometimes is called as the mask of pregnancy! The nipples should also get progressively darker throughout the pregnancy, which is caused by the hormonal changes that produce more pigment in the skin, in that case in the areolas – the skin around the nipples. The round ligaments of the abdomen are stretching where some abdominal achiness may be experienced, and the pelvic joints are loosening up to allow the uterus' growth.

Food cravings and increased appetite can also increase the physical body weight, and in combination with the growing womb and the extra weight on the front of the torso could unbalance the center of body gravity, which in turn can cause clumsiness and also strain the lumbar region as the muscles work on keeping the body balanced. Dizziness, headaches and mild edema in the limbs is common even in a healthy pregnancy, as the blood pressure is lowered naturally by hormones secreted to accommodate the extra need for fluids to the placenta. Considering the extra weight gained with the low blood pressure and the slowed blood circulation, a woman can start experiencing cramps, develop fluid retention in the limbs and/or face and varicose veins.

Piles is also common in pregnancy and usually start appearing on the second trimester. These happen because hormones make the veins relaxed, and then clusters of veins in rectum or anus get swollen or dilated. Constipation starts appearing at this trimester and can continue until the end of pregnancy, and this occurs for two reasons; because of iron supplement intake, and because the colon and intestines are squeezed to give more room to the growing uterus. Similarly, the whole digestive system is squeezed and the woman can have heartburn, indigestion, flatulence, frequent urination.

Hormonal changes during the pregnancy can make gums swollen or sore that can cause bleeding. These hormonal changes cause healthy hair and nails' growth because of higher estrogen levels, however, if androgens are higher than normal, may result in facial and body hair growth as well.

Thinking of the woman's mental state, this is the trimester she realizes the pregnancy and starts having worries and anxiety about baby's healthy and safe development, and also starts thinking of childbirth. Her general concentration level can be decreased and her emotions become unstable as she develops irritability, weepiness, anxiety, moodiness, happiness, joy, excitement!

What is important to remember is that many women will start practicing yoga from this trimester onwards. The pregnancy effects of nausea, vomiting and fatigue, and the risk of miscarriage is usually gone at the second trimester which can make the mother-to-be more energetic and joyful. We, as prenatal yoga teachers, should make sure they do not overstrain themselves during practical sessions. Due to the increased energy levels, it is common for pregnant ladies to push the yoga teacher to push them to more strenuous practices. In such cases you should always consider every practitioner as a separate case where you should be opening each class by discussing possible aches and pregnancy symptoms. It is advisable to plan you class sequence in a way you always include hip and chest opening asanas, as well as those for strengthening and relieving lower back pain. Also, sleeping difficulty usually starts at the second trimester, and neck/ shoulders issues appear from bad posture and pressure on the vertebrae, therefore asanas helping these fields will make practitioners more rejuvenated and confident.

Specific focus should be given on teaching practitioners on modifications, while they can still feel relieved from stretching by having their full awareness and acknowledgment on their constant changing body. Although it is not required for us pre-postnatal yoga teachers to have in depth anatomical and physiological knowledge, it is our duty to understand how the pregnant body develops. This will help us protect our students from injuries or accidents and at the same time teach a well-balanced class.

As a mandra for a practitioner on her second trimester, even if she can still sit on Base Position – Prarambhik Sthiti with legs closed to practice asanas, such asanas must be performed with legs open to the edges of the mat. While on second and third trimester, we emphasize sitting with opened legs and accommodating the belly nicely and comfortably with stretched legs open, because if one is sitting with closed legs, there is a natural compression at the lower part of the belly which we need to avoid at this stage of pregnancy. The purpose of especially prenatal practices is to open front hip area and the whole genital and pelvic floor area. Sitting with opened legs while practicing, benefits the natural pull in the inner thigh, in the groin area, along with the cervix that gets stimulated when legs are open and helps entering into a healthy labor period. If at this stage of pregnancy, a woman is sitting with closed legs, then she may experience difficulties in hip opening, in inner thigh stretch, as well as difficulty opening up the birth canal in the cervix area. To achieve the same as the pregnancy progresses to the third trimester, the mother-to-be should be on Base Position with her legs as wide open as it feels comfortable and outside of the mat.

When entering the second trimester, it is important to focus more on strengthening the legs and hip opening, as the pregnant body needs to start preparing for labor. Standing asanas and balanced ones are beneficial for leg strengthening and also help preventing edema or swelling in the lower limbs, as they increase blood circulation. When practicing wide-legged standing poses, such as Warrior II – Virabhadrasana II, need to be aware of the pelvic floor which is already strained, therefore it is advisable to either reduce the width of the legs or practice seated on a chair.

Any prone positioning should be totally avoided until after childbirth. Any abdominal practices such as Boat Pose – Naukasana or leg lifts such Pawanmuktasana Part 2 and 3 should be completely avoided, as the abdominal muscles and ligaments start stretching to accommodate the growing belly and there is danger of muscle separation or tear. The Padmasana group of asanas should not be practiced during pregnancy as the blood circulation in the legs is reduced. Inverted and backward bending asanas are also not recommended during pregnancy, apart from Kandharasana or Setu Bandha Sarvangasana that will give the benefits of backward bends and Parvatasana which can be practiced with ease and normal breathing. Any twists have to be modified so the move happens above the waist and should be gentle and not too deep to help release the lumbar area.

- Chair Pose – Utkatasana

- Extended Side Angle Pose – Utthita Parsvakonasana

- Extended Triangle Pose – Utthita Trikonasana

- Goddess Pose – Kaliasana

- Half Moon Pose – Ardha Chandrasana

- Lizard Pose – Utthan Pristhasana

- One-Legged Prayer or Tree Pose – Eka Pada Pranamasana

- Reverse Warrior Pose – Viparita Virabhadrasana

- Warrior I – Virabhadrasana I

- Warrior II – Virabhadrasana II

The muscles in the upper back region take the extra weight of the breasts, so Gomukhasana can help release this tension. From week 20 onwards, the mother-to-be should avoid any supine positioning, but if she does, that should last only for a minute or two to the maximum. Instead of Shavasana, practitioner could be on a modified Matsya Kridasana lying on the left side and not on the stomach, so not to put pressure to the belly, but also importantly to avoid compressing the inferior vena cava – the major vein carrying blood from lower body, back to uterus and the heart. This compression is caused by the weight of the uterus and growing baby, leading to reduced amount of blood return. It is recommended to use blankets, cushions, pillows or a bolster under the right knee, right arm and head so she is fully supported and comfortable. additionally, you can guide your students to reclining poses that will increase blood circulation to the legs, will open up the hips and relieve back pain. It is strongly advisable to use blankets, cushions, pillows or a bolster to elevate upper body at around 20° or 30° degrees.

- Extended Supine Hand to Big Toe Pose – Utthita Supta Padangusthasana

- Reclined Butterfly Pose – Supta Baddhakonasana

- Side-Reclining Leg Lift Pose – Anantasana

- Sleeping Thunderbolt Pose – Supta Vajrasana

Modifications should be introduced for most of the asanas hereafter, including the folded or twisted ones. On forward bends the practitioner should open the legs slightly and bend from the hips, while at the same time she has her full awareness not to compress the abdomen area and her growing belly. On spinal twisting asanas, only the open twists are advised to be practiced, which can equally release back pain and nicely stretch the body. All twisting should be from above the waist and should not be too deep, with full awareness again not to compress the abdomen area and growing belly.

- Airplane Pose – Kati Sakti Vikasaka

- Back Stretching Pose – Paschimottanasana

- Swaying Palm Tree Pose – Tiryak Tadasana

Pranayama and Yoga Nidra should be continued or introduced if not practicing already, to help in balancing emotions, remove stress and anxiety, calm the body and mind. For until the end of second trimester, pranayama is beneficial for both mother and baby, as baby's lungs are not yet fully formed and totally depends on prana source from the mother. Ocean or Psychic Breath – Ujjayi Pranayama is a good practice that can also help during labor and delivery. Any pranayama technique with breath retention or flow of air alteration, such as Kapalbhati (Frontal Brain Cleansing or Skull Shining Breath) should be totally avoided as the prana source – the delivery of oxygen to the fetus, will be disturbed. On the other hand, Yoga Nidra is important for relaxation, energy boosting and also helping mother to connect with her baby. By the fifth month the baby becomes more active inside the womb and mother can start feeling these movements. When mother is on a relaxation pose, yoga nidra can encourage a mental and physical connection of mother and baby.

It is important to keep reminding your students the importance of resting and relaxation after any type of physical practice. During your practical sessions you can train your students on certain Mantra. Practicing these at home at their own relaxation time will help enhancing energy flow, focus and concentration.

The Pregnant Body – Third Trimester

The timeframe for third trimester is between 29-40 weeks of pregnancy and is the last and final stage of pregnancy. Many women at this trimester worry about their gained weight and should always keep in mind that average baby's weight at childbirth in 40 weeks is between 2.5 to 4 kg (5,5 to 8,8 pounds; 88 to 141 ounces), and the extra weight from the support fluids that keep the baby healthy and alive weights approximately 6.2 kg (13,6 pounds; 218 ounces).

The extra weight a woman has put on during her pregnancy other than the actual baby weight and support system, can cause great discomfort especially towards the end of the pregnancy. Food cravings and the increased appetite with no balanced nutrition can increase her weight which can also contribute to her stressing out. The enlargement, soreness and tenderness of breasts with possible leaking of colostrum, a precursor to milk, especially towards the end and the larger womb can create discomfort and difficulty in moving and sleeping. The uterus is getting extra pressure from the growing baby that can result in short breath, lower back pain or sciatica. The internal organs are also getting extra pressure that can cause short breath, heartburn, indigestion, flatulence, frequent urination, and constipation especially in combination with iron supplements' intake. Occasional dizziness or faintness as well as swelling/ edema may be experienced because of the progesterone hormone which slows down blood circulation and can cause fluid retention in upper and lower limbs and/or face. The relaxin hormone makes the joints unstable and sensitive, however it is useful to prepare pelvis for labor and childbirth.

The baby may begin to move into the lower abdomen and with baby's weight development extra pressure will be put on the bladder which may lead to hemorrhoids' development for the mother-to-be. Especially in cases of aggravated hemorrhoids, avoid giving deep squatting practices as the pressure will be even more and create more discomfort.

From the seventh month, depending the woman's lifestyle, she may experience decreased energy and fatigue, or increased energy. She should be feeling baby's movements by now and as her belly grows, she might have abdominal achiness as uterus stretches, and as the pregnancy progresses she might be having an itchy belly. She might also start feeling heaviness of the abdomen. From the eighth month, the pregnant body starts getting prepared for the labor and childbirth. Braxton-Hicks contractions or periodic tightening of the uterine muscles will be felt, as these muscle contractions are vital for vaginal childbirth, whereas towards the end of the ninth month these contractions will be becoming more intense and frequent. By the middle of ninth month, the baby should have taken positioning, which can make walking, sitting and standing up more difficult than usual. The cervix also starts dilating and as the pelvic floor gradually softens up until labor, the water breaks which indicate the baby is ready to emerge to this world.

During this trimester, it is very common for the woman to experience insomnia, caused either by her physical body discomfort or by excess thinking of the future. Thinking and dreaming about a healthy and safe baby from childbirth to growth into adulthood is a process women develop naturally from pregnancy period.

While practicing yoga, it is always important to remember that with the growing womb, whether a woman feels comfortable and active or tired, in pain and with possible mobility issues, yogic practices have to be modified accordingly. For those who tend to preterm labor or complications most asanas and specifically squatting must be avoided. Yoga is safe and can be practiced until the day the woman goes into labor, even during labor, and practicing should always be done with full care and awareness for safety. However, it is the time to give more emphasis on pranayama techniques and less on asanas to encourage relaxation and concentration. Can be practiced either on its own; or during relaxation; or in a favorite hip-opening pose such as Child's Pose – Shashankasana with the support of pillows or cushions supporting the knees; or while practicing to enhance focus. Yoga Nidra, Meditation, visualization, mantra and chanting can enhance the emotional balance and ease the possible fears the mother-to-be may be having either for the childbirth process and/or the future.

Throughout the second and third trimester, hip opening practices are most important as they assist in releasing the lumbar spine and relieving any aches and also open up the pelvic region and hip joints to prepare the body for labor. Pelvic tilts have a dual benefit, as by lifting they tone up and by lowering they soften up the pelvic floor, while squatting and Cat and Cow Stretch Pose – Marjariasana encourage proper baby positioning in the uterus – head down facing the back.

- Back Stretching Pose – Paschimottanasana

- Extended Puppy Pose – Uttana Shishosana

- Full Butterfly – Poorna Titali Asana

- Half Forward Bend – Ardha Uttanasana

- Salutation Pose – Namaskarsana

- Seated Cat & Cow Pose – Marjariasana

- Spiraled Head to Knee Pose – Parivritti Janu Sirshasana

- Wide Angled Seated Forward Bend – Upavistha Konasana

Asanas that promote relaxation and strength should be practicing more frequently now so the pregnant body get prepared for labor and childbirth. Focusing on protecting the joints and maintaining balance is equally important as the extra weight the mother-to-be is carrying – in combination with the growing belly, creates difficulty to balance the center of her gravity. Basic standing and balancing asanas are good to be practiced (with the support of a wall or a chair or a table to secure balance) for strengthening the legs, maintaining proper spinal alignment and encouraging blood circulation.

- Chair Pose – Utkatasana

- Duck Walking – Karandavasana

- Extended Side Angle Pose – Utthita Parsvakonasana

- Extended Triangle Pose – Utthita Trikonasana

- Legs Up The Wall Pose – Viparita Karani

- One-Legged Prayer or Tree Pose – Eka Pada Pranamasana

- Reverse Warrior Pose – Viparita Virabhadrasana

- Warrior I – Virabhadrasana I

- Warrior II – Virabhadrasana II

Pranayama can also work as a guide for possible challenging poses, such as the Eka Pada Pranamasana, in which the practitioner can shift her positioning by following her breath and body capacity, without coming out of the pose. She can take short breaks in between the sequence to get to the pose while she maintains a smooth breath work.

The Postnatal Body – Fourth Trimester

The changes in a woman's body during pregnancy, childbirth and postnatal period are enormous. Her internal organs are naturally moving to accommodate the necessary needs, her hormones are unbalanced during the pre and postnatal period, the childbirth has shocked the body, which all affect her physical and mental state of being.

Emotionally

A woman's body has gone through a lot during her pregnancy, as well as the body sock during labor. If a woman had "baby blues" before childbirth (i.e. crying for no particular reason, mood swings, anxiety or insomnia), it is likely to experience Postpartum Depression. For all these emotional changes is mostly the hormones to blame! The estrogen and progesterone were higher during pregnancy, while after childbirth these drop dramatically. Also the endorphins released by hypothalamus and pituitary gland can make a woman feel happy or even stressed or depressed. There are women who feel insecure, anxious or even panic in presence of their crying baby, stressing themselves between what feels right and what is known to be right so far. Yoga nidra, asanas, pranayama can all help balance the emotions and prevent postpartum depression.

To help increase body's endorphins one can practice asanas when healthcare advisor has approved doing so, but before that, it is absolutely safe to practice Pranayama, Yoga Nidra, Mantra and Chanting during the fourth trimester. These will bring balance and calmness to the emotions and also recharge and give energy to the new mum. Along with releasing endorphins, exercising, meditating, listening to favorite music, exposing oneself to the direct sun, bonding with the newborn and the rest of the family, breastfeeding, laughing and feeling love can also alter levels of serotonin and dopamine which all can boost up the emotional being of a new mother.

Physically

For the mother to start practicing asanas, all depend on delivery type. There is a usual 6-week checkup post-delivery in which the health advisor will have to confirm when practice can consume, depending on the delivery type – normal delivery, episiotomy, caesarean section, and any interventions – tearing or stiches. In all cases other than caesarean section, there is discomfort on the genital area during the healing period and practicing any asanas during this time should be totally avoided. Usually, gentle practicing can start 6 or 7 weeks after childbirth, and 3 months later a regular yoga routine can be consumed. Kegel exercises can be practiced much earlier if the woman feels right to do so, but there should be no hip or pelvic opening practices during the fourth trimester. As soon as body has healed, Bhujangasana, Parsva Balasana, Marjariasana, and mild practices can be re-introduced. In episiotomy, there should be no Half or Full Butterfly practicing until stiches have dropped and wound has completely healed.

In the case of C-section, there should be a waiting for at least 8 weeks or longer if the wound has not healed completely, and usually 6 months later a regular yoga routine can be practiced. After a C-section, a woman has been through a major abdominal surgery and is normal to feel pain in that area, soreness and possible bleeding. In either case, the C-Section wound or any tearing or stitching must be treated with care and according to the healthcare provider's guidelines. Usually such skin stiches take up to 3 weeks to dissolve, however, underlying stiches in the muscle layer will take a little longer to fully heal. The healthcare advisor has to confirm timeframe and suggest types of practices according to practitioners' body healing. Any prone asanas are not allowed.

Lochia bleeding is normal for up to 6 weeks, as the uterus sheds its lining. If lochia bleeding exceeds the sixth or seventh week, it is recommended to consult the healthcare provider.

For those who had piles during pregnancy (either internal and/or external), they may carry on having them for a few more days.

Incontinence of urine or frequent urination will gradually resolve after a few weeks or a few months. If haven't been already practicing Kegel exercises to tighten pelvic floor muscles, it is a good time to start doing so, especially if had a normal delivery with no complications.

It is hormonal to experience healthy hair and nails' growth during pregnancy because of higher estrogen levels. It is also normal after childbirth, to experience hair loss and nails breakage caused by falling estrogen levels. This is only temporary, and one need to be aware that people loose hair for many reasons, however if hair loss is a worrying sign, one may always consult a Dermatologist for an accurate diagnosis and effective personalized treatment.

Breast changes are common and natural during and after childbirth. After childbirth, breasts produce colostrum first, which is highly nutritious as it is rich in antibodies for the infant and higher in protein, fat, carbohydrates, magnesium, vitamins A, B, C and E and minerals than any other form of milk. After a few days, milk is secreted by prolactin hormone (from pituitary gland) and somatomammotropin (from the placenta). Breasts may be enlarged now as they are full and may feel them tender and hot. The nipples may be becoming sensitive during the first days of breastfeeding and may be experiencing some pain on that area during nursing; it is normal at this stage. After a few days, nipple hardens and the pain goes gradually. The Ayurvedic and Yogic approach to treat sensitive nipples is application of ghee; and for sore breasts and better blood circulation it is recommended to massage them with mustard oil, starting from areola and upward chest movements.

Practicing yoga post-delivery is important because it tones up the core and abdominal muscles, helps the uterus come back to its original shape and position, promotes a fast recovery and improves overall well-being. Therefore, during the fourth trimester, specific focus should be given on strengthening the pelvic floor, abdominal muscles, lower back and toning the uterus.

In the first month after childbirth, focus more on pranayama to rest the body, and also balance body and mind. To release tensions from neck, shoulders, ankles and improve blood circulation, one can practice gentle joint movements from Pawanmuktasana Part 1.

When healthcare advisor has confirmed the woman's well-being and asanas are allowed to be gently consumed, specific focus should be given on strengthening the pelvic floor, abdominal muscles, lumbar area and toning the uterus, as well as closing the pelvic floor. Any pelvic opening practices should be totally avoided during this time. Stretching the shoulders, upper back and neck, opening the chest (to improve lactation), improving posture and releasing tension in these areas are considered safe for practice.

Although the abdomen is soft and flabby, labor, breastfeeding and lack of sleep can make body tense and stiff which leads to low energy levels and fatigue. Kegels, simple neck stretches and shoulder rotations can release tension from the specific areas and can be performed as early as it feels right to do so. It is also important to consider spanx for postpartum belly as soon as possible, to help the postnatal body reduce back and pelvic floor pain, support posture, encourage blood flow, provide additional compression to help recovering abdominal muscles, even from a C-section or diastasis recti.

- Camel Pose – Ushtrasana

- Cat and Cow Stretch Pose – Marjariasana

- Cobra Pose – Bhujangasana

- Cow's Face Pose – Gomukhasana

- Hero's Meditation Pose – Dhyana Veerasana

- Legs Up The Wall Pose – Viparita Karani

- Sun Salutation – Surya Namaskar

- Swaying Palm Tree Pose – Tiryak Tadasana

Embryonic Development

As a prenatal yoga teacher you don't need to know everything about how a baby develops. However, some basic knowledge can help you connect with your students. Having some general knowledge of when baby's heart begins to beat or by when a would-be-mum starts feeling her baby's moves or having general anatomy knowledge of baby's 'home' in mum's womb, can help you connect better with your students. Discussions about what they are experiencing become more efficient and that will give you're a better understanding on how they are feeling.

Herein, baby's development is broken down into three trimesters, presenting basic information.

Weeks 1-12

From a fertilized egg the first 12 weeks is a time with rapid development for the baby.

By week 4 the nervous system, brain, spinal cord and heart have begun to form. Arms and leg buds begin to develop and is now an embryo.

By week 6, the embryo is 13-16mm long and the heart has started to beat. The brain, stomach and intestines are developing.

By week 7-8, the embryo begins to develop into a fetus and all major organs have begun to form. Arms and legs are growing longer, fingers and toes are about to begin forming. Sex organs also start forming at this time.

By the end of week 12 – First Trimester, the fetus is approximately 11cm long and weights around 45gr. All the organs have formed and heart beat is audible with a Doppler.

Weeks 13-28

By week 16, the fetus is approximately 18cm long, weights around 200gr and the circulatory and urinary system are functioning. Sex organs are fully formed and parents-to-be can find out the sex of the baby if they desire so.

By week 18-20, the fetus' heart beat is often detectable with a stethoscope and would-be-mum can start to feel baby move.

By week 24, the baby is approximately 31cm long and weights around 700gr. The skin is covered in fine hair, protected with a waxy coating and the taste buds are forming. Baby can now recognize mum's voice.

By the end of week 28 – Second Trimester, the baby is approximately 36cm long and weights around 1100gr. The hair, nails, eyebrows and eyelashes have completed formed, the eyelids have opened and the lungs have grown enough to be able to breathe outside the uterus with medical support. The ears and hearing is fully developed.

Weeks 29-40

During the third trimester, baby will not only be gaining weight quickly, but also its' brain develops rapidly.

By week 32, the baby is approximately 41cm long, weights around 1800gr and is inhaling amniotic fluid to exercise its lungs and practice breathing.

By week 36, the baby weights around 2600gr and gains weight rapidly every week and grows faster which helps baby to be born healthy, as such, may be having limited movement inside the womb due to restricted space. It can be considered as full term and can be born anytime from then on without been classed as premature.

By week 40 – the due date, the baby may be approximately 50cm and weight around 3200gr.

Baby's Home

Amniotic Sac: Baby is growing and developing inside the amniotic sac, a bag of amniotic fluid that lines the inside of the uterus. The amniotic fluid nourishes and protects the baby and averages 800ml at about 34th week of gestation, where at week 40 averages 600ml.

Placenta: During pregnancy, the pregnant body develops an organ, the placenta, to provide baby with nutrients and oxygen and removes waste products from baby's blood.

Mucus Plug: The mucus plug is a protective mass of mucus in the cervical canal. This collection of mucus is formed in early pregnancy to protect the fetus and later baby against bacteria or any other form of infection. It is normal for the would-be-mum to lose the mucus plug as she reaches closer to full term and the cervix prepares for labor.

Pregnancy Guidelines

During pregnancy the body changes, and for those willing to yog, they need to follow certain guidelines for the safety of the pregnancy and the unborn baby. During this time, yoga should not be practiced in the same way as it was during the pre-conception period of a woman's life, and should definitely be practiced for the benefits of both would-be-mum's and baby's healthy development. At this time, anything new and advanced should be avoided. The woman needs to be gentle and caring for both herself and her unborn baby. An experienced and trained teacher can always guide the class through safety and relaxation. Breathing techniques in coordination with the asana practice, as well as the awareness of every asana can benefit the physical movement, the breathing itself, raise concentration on a specific area. Chakras function better and get activated as these are associated with the nerve plexuses and the endocrine glands in the body, if we talk about physical awareness; and if we talk about spiritual awareness, each chakra is defining a specific part/ organ of the body and when awareness is moved to that point during asanas, the benefits can only increase.

✘ As a principle, there should be no belly compression, strain or overstretching. Overstretching can occur itself due to relaxin hormone increase, which softens the muscles and ligaments.

✘ Avoid strong twists; instead practice gentle open ones.

✘ Avoid Abdominal practices, especially after second trimester. May experience abdominal contractions and as pregnancy progresses may give false alarms for Braxton Hicks contractions. Any strain on the pelvic area, especially during the first trimester may harm pregnancy. Exercises such as (heavy) weight lifting, strong gym practicing and while yoga practicing, intense abdominal core strengthening poses such as Boat Pose – Naukasana are not to be practiced. Similar poses in yoga with both legs raised, such as Locust or Fish Pose with raised legs should be generally avoided; even Half Boat pose with the knees raised is an intense upper abdominal core pose will also put unnecessary pelvic floor pressure at this time.

✘ Gentle Backbends and modified ones can benefit body aches and stretch the spine and the back during pregnancy, however, as the pregnancy progresses there can be more curvature on the lower back and in this case backbends should be practiced with extra care. Strong backbends are not recommended throughout a pregnancy.

✘ Avoid any Prone poses even from the first trimester if there is breast tenderness, certainly from second trimester onwards.

✘ Avoid Supine poses at any stage of pregnancy if it feels uncomfortable or causes dizziness or faintness. Reason for these symptoms is the compression to Vena Cava, the main vein returning blood to the heart from the lower extremities and abdomen. Pressure on the vein can decrease oxygen supply to both mother and baby. Additionally, if need to be on supine position, choose to lie down on left side which can increase oxygen supply. Generally, it is recommended to totally avoid supine poses from 34th week onwards.

✘ Avoid Inverted poses as these may put extra pressure on the inferior vena cava and lead to dizziness. Especially after 32nd week any inverted pose must be avoided as this is the time for baby to prepare for birth and get into position.

✘ Avoid Holding poses and pranayama for extended time. When exercising holding Standing poses can be demanding for your breath capacity and current body abilities. The pulse rate increases with any type of exercise, and when practicing holding poses even for 15-20 counts the heart is working a lot harder than usual which can lead to over-exhaustion. Moreover, holding for too long can decrease blood flow to the uterus and cause dizziness and venous pooling, which is increased blood pressure in leg veins that don't allow correct blood circulation.

✘ Avoid Squatting if there are complications in the pregnancy.

✘ Must be cautious when moving from Supine to Sitting poses and from Sitting to Standing and vice versa. Such moves should always be done carefully and gently and especially from supine positioning should roll to the left side before slowly sitting up. That way dizziness may be decreased at that time and also there will be no stress on lower back, belly or the abdominal muscles and pelvic area.

Although every pregnancy is different, all poses should feel comfortable and there should be no strain or over-exertion. Any pose that feels uncomfortable or just not right, breathless or experience increased heart rate just release this at once. When practicing yoga asanas during pregnancy should focus on creating space and openness. Following steady and comfortable poses with additional care will help to enjoy yoga and only benefit from it!

Prenatal Care

Prenatal care is important to encourage mother's and baby's health and well-being. It is always advisable to visit the healthcare provider from the moment she realizes pregnancy or even when she thinks she is carrying. The doctor or midwife will be able to identify possible issues that might affect her own health and pregnancy itself. Regular visits and check-ups as per healthcare provider's request should be followed thoroughly as any possible problems can be spotted and treated at an early stage. Especially if the mother-to-be is having a high risk pregnancy, carrying twins, or is new to fitness, and in her late pregnancy if the baby is breech, she must consult her healthcare advisor before practicing any type of exercise.

The Pregnancy Guidelines as explained on previous chapter should be remembered and followed for a safe practice. Yoga should be helping everyone and especially an expecting woman to feel peaceful and relaxed and should be a joyful time.

Not all pregnancies are normal; there are high risk and low risk pregnancies. Whether you are experiencing one or as yoga teacher you need to cue for your students, you need to understand the complications. In this book we will identify the most common pregnancy complications and will point practices to help each of the symptoms. Understanding the complications and treating them is the healthcare provider's duty; understanding the complications as confident or as experienced a yoga teacher may be, is always good to consult a physician for advice before starting to cue prenatal classes. If you are running or planning to run a pre-postnatal studio, it may be an asset for your business to have such a healthcare professional linked to your business. That professional can provide physiological guidance to you and your students, which will lead to more relaxed and confident practices. We, yoga professionals have no intention to harm anyone (Ahimsa), however, on a high-risk pregnancy we don't want to take the extra risk! We care for the well-being of our client and the life she carries inside her womb!

Healthy eating and prenatal diet and nutrition in general is a trend nowadays on every phase of our lives. Eating right during pregnancy can lead to a healthy pregnancy and a healthy baby.

Yogic Guidelines for Labor and Birthing

Yoga helps a woman to be physically, mentally and spiritually prepared for labor and birthing. This is a major event in every woman's life that is a very emotional and physical event, which transforms a woman for life. Whichever is the plan for birthing, i.e. natural or caesarian, yoga trains the woman to be relaxed and calm during the process, which relaxation and calmness is automatically transferred to the baby. It is important for the baby to experience this peace coming from the mother, to enter the physical world in its first moments of life with happy first feelings. During pre-labor and labor, there might be complications for which the obstetrician should decide if an episiotomy may be required or a caesarian section for mother's and baby health. It doesn't matter which is the way, as long as there is a safe and healthy birthing. We should be grateful for the wonderful pregnancy journey and be prepared to continue nurturing with care and love our baby for the rest of our lives.

What needs to be noted before birth and during labor is that the woman's body is perfectly designed in terms of anatomy, physiology and energy to nurture a life during pregnancy and give birth. Women have been doing this since the beginning of time and every woman should have faith in herself, the universe and the marvelous female energy. Birth is a natural miracle and every woman should feel lucky and grateful for this experience and gift, and should trust her own body's and baby's ability to constant growth, wisdom, and power to develop. With every contraction there is a cervical expansion and should keep as calm and relaxed as possible, as this natural process will lead to birthing. All pain that comes with it, can be considered as tension in the body which is vital to help baby move out. If the woman has the courage to experience birthing by observing and embracing it, by noticing sensations, practice pranayama techniques or even chanting or what may make her feel better, she will come to realize the pain works with her and should welcome it. The energy of birthing comes from the woman and her baby, therefore she should accept it and surrender to it with trust for a healthy and quick childbirth. One should avoid reading or hearing negative stories on childbirth, these apply only to special occasions and are not the rule; trust your body and self, trust your healthcare advisor. Focus on the positive affirmations, thinking and practices for a mental and physical health. On the final stages of labor, it may be helpful to practice visualization techniques, such as *"I am opening up like a flower opens up"*. This could help divert the thought process from labor pain to a wonderful sensation and ease the pain.

Breathing

During labor there is not a particular yogic breathing technique one should follow, however, deep relaxed breathing is recommended while trying to bring awareness on the breath to divert mind from pain. Everyone should be conscious of how much energy is in the breath and its power. With every inhalation we are riving prana, balance, oxygen to our system. With every exhalation we release tensions, stress, anxiety and anything negative. By feeling and witnessing the breath will help stay focused and relaxed to a certain level during labor. Attempt to bring awareness on breathing downward as well as focusing on the abdomen and baby can also help the birthing process.

An experienced yoga practitioner may be able to focus on breathing and practice pranayama techniques that can be helpful:

Yogic Breath while visualizing a flower opening at the cervical region. Visualization directs mind from pain. Ujjayi Pranayama, benefits during and between contractions as it can help to relax, center and connect with the breathing and birthing process. Bhramari, benefits on releasing natural endorphins for pain relief, and the sound has healing effects which can also help to connect with inner strength.

Chanting & Sounds

During childbirth, there are women who have the need to make sounds, while other remain silent. It is a very personal thing, that works differently between individuals. Chanting Om, or other sounds like 'Aaa' or 'Mmm' can be helpful for connecting to own self for inner strength. Those who can't chant can also consider having an audio to listen Om chanting or other mantra chants of their choice. The soothing and calming effects of chanting when surrendering to the sounds can only be great during childbirth! And the baby, coming out to our physically world has these first experiences of sounds to calm from the transition of being inside the womb and the birthing experience!

Asanas

With the use of a strong heavy item such as a bed, the wall or a partner for support can practice any combination of the following asanas, which all focus on opening the pelvis, help dilation, encourage optimal baby position to navigate through the pelvis and descend.

- ✓ Squatting practices

- ✓ Standing and bending slightly forward.

- ✓ Kneeling on the bed or on a soft yoga mat.

- ✓ Half Kneeling, thinking of a kneeled warrior, in which one knee is on the ground and the other foot is on the ground.

- ✓ Marjariasana helps on back pain management, and if can place awareness to connect breath and rocking movement can achieve rhythm and relaxation. Can be practiced with the palms of the hands on the ground or on forearms.

- ✓ Anantasana with the support of cushions under the belly. Raising and bending one leg, or modified Matsya Kridasana with support of pillows or bolster to keep knees steady and comfortable to the hips level. These asanas are helpful for the baby to get through the pelvis, especially if it is in Occiput Posterior (OP) position[1]. The Matsya Kridasana can be mostly beneficial to those who can't move around.

- ✓ Poorna Titali Asana benefits in the early stages of labor and those who had an epidural and are restricted to bed.

- ✓ Ardha Uttanasana the variation leaning forward to a wall for stretching can also take pressure off woman's lower back.

- ✓ Shashankasana with the support of cushions or a Pilates ball to hug on if practiced between contractions can offer relaxation. In that pose can also practice pelvic rotations.

Although this is not an asana, place your hands on the belly to send loving thoughts and connect with the baby and your energies. Labor is a painful experience for the woman, but also a stressing one for the baby.

---

[1] Baby's head is downward position, but instead of facing back it is facing the front.

Post-Natal Yoga

There are many who will come and tell about the extra weight and a woman's body changes after childbirth, but most of them neglect the fact that this woman has just gave birth to another life and her body has gone through major emotional and physical changes. The pressure many women experience in handling all the changes in their life is enormous, especially if someone considers they might still be in pain, let along their body naturally needs approximately 9 to 12 months to fully recover. In the pain list we could add sleepless days and nights, malnutrition, stress to connect and find quality time with her other children and partner, feeling loneliness and isolation, which all may lead to anxiety. People mostly care about what they see, and the Postnatal period is a time when everyone is praising the newborn and many stress out the mother with questions about her extra weight. All it matters is that simple questions can irritate a new mother, and her hormones, character and fatigue are all struggling to balance the new her; postpartum depression!

Yoga Teachers specializing in Pre and Postnatal Yoga, we are trained and certified to deal with such cases. Exercise in general and Yoga in particular release dopamine, oxytocin, serotonin and endorphin hormones which help lower stress levels and anxiety and work to benefit calmness, relaxation and manage body weight.

Motherhood Yoga – The First Year

Motherhood in the first year can be difficult and challenging for many. Conceiving, carrying and giving birth to a baby is a gift of life and all women should be grateful! That gives them the power to cherish and unconditionally love the life around them! Regardless, motherhood is a hard and at the same time wonderful 24/7 job, where all experience physical and emotional changes.

For the breastfeeding mums, especially for the first 6 months, it seems like breastfeeding is the only commitment they have, which changes as soon as baby is introduced to solid food. For some women, breastfeeding is a loving process, for some other a difficult and uncomfortable one. For the women who can't breastfeed their babies due to organic difficulties, it can cause anxiety and negative emotions towards themselves or their baby. It is possible to feel guilt, anger, sadness or even depression. Yogic practices when combined can help boost the emotional state, energy levels and also sustain and increase milk production.

Certain asanas, pranayama, relaxation and Om chanting can be done even during breastfeeding, benefiting both mother and baby. Yoga Nidra can help recharge, rejuvenate and relax everyone, and for those women who are lacking sleep, it will give them the feeling and energy of a few hours' sleep.

For someone to start teaching or self-practicing yoga after childbirth, needs to be aware of the postnatal body. Any practice for any duration in time during breastfeeding should be with caution, because the body is in a state of physical and energetic openness. Further to that, there are women who have diastasis recti and sacro-iliac misalignments post birth, as well as those who delivered with a caesarean section which is considered as a surgery, therefore, the focus should be closing and strengthening the physical body. Any wide opening asanas and overstretching is not advisable. A woman in lactation needs to know that breastfeeding extends the levels of relaxin in the body, causing softness and flabbiness which is normal. Even if she is still on lochia, had episiotomy or C-section, until the end of fourth trimester, it is advisable for her to only practice a nice warm-up routine, such as the Pawanmuktasana Part 1, unless her healthcare advisor suggests differently. She can easily practice these asanas while lying on her bed or seated in a chair. If she feels comfortable and have recovered from lochia, pains, stitching or tearing, she can practice these while standing with the support of a wall if needed, or on her mat.

For practicing postnatal yoga, we have two timeframes to consider. The timeframe from childbirth and the timeframe of breastfeeding. In the timeframe from childbirth we consider the body recovery duration depending of the delivery type (C-section, episiotomy, normal delivery, tearing, or stitching); the main changes and common problems in the physical and mental level; and the endocrine system and how this works for breastfeeding and non-breastfeeding women. In the breastfeeding timeframe which is decided solely by mother and baby alone, practice should be with ease and with modifications, similarly to the prenatal duration. While on breastfeeding period, the woman should practice with the use of props on any prone position, such as pillows or cushions, as a support system between her breasts and the ground, and that should last for as long as she feels her breasts full and hard, approximately 4 to 6 months. When practicing, mindfulness is the mantra to avoid any potential risk from overstretching and excessive practice to come back to her fitness, as her lactation may be affected in quality and quantity, at some times may be even stopped. Therefore, the asanas she can practice should be easy, comfortable and not forceful at all.

The main focus in the postnatal period is to ease the upper body stiffness which is caused by bad body posture while breastfeeding, as well as tone up the lower limb and side abdomen and waist area. For a woman just now starting to consume her yoga asanas after childbirth, even with a small pain or tearing during the yoga practice, she should stop at once and allow herself one more week of rest. Because we have to work with a sensitive body of a woman in her post-delivery period, we as yoga teachers are no doctors – unless one possesses such qualifications, our knowledge comes from practicing yoga, and although human anatomy studies we had, gave us a clear and detailed understanding of how prenatal and postnatal body functions, it is always recommended to seek for healthcare advisor's approval before starting regular yoga routines.

From my personal experience, the job of a non-breastfeeding mum is the most difficult one. Having personally non-breastfed my first born son, and years later breastfed my daughter, I can certainly relate to both experiences and also share that people treat the woman differently only by considering the way she feeds her baby. For us yoga teachers, the differentiation between the ways a newborn can be fed arises solely from the selection of asanas and their benefits for the mother alone. For the non-breastfeeding mother, the fact she feeds her baby by the bottle, doesn't mean her body is recovering faster. Her body reacts in the exact same physical way to recover from childbirth as any other woman, but for her, the endocrine system and secreted hormones will control her moods and emotions and may need more time to balance.

She can easily practice the asanas given for a breastfeeding mum, however, a special focus should be given on selecting asanas to help her emotionally as she may be experiencing anxiety for her inability to breastfeed her baby, or even suffer postpartum depression and also importantly tone up her body. At this phase of her life, a woman needs to start feeling confident, and her physical body appearance play a key role to her emotional state of being. Her body is also stiff, whether she breastfeeds or nurses with a bottle.

As the baby grows day-by-day, the baby weight increases, the body posture is lucking attention, she is most probably missing meals and sleep to catch up with everything, and all these lead to body stiffness and fatigue. Although her physical body may be ready for consuming exercise, through yoga practicing we do not want to cause further exhaustion. Our aim is to relieve her pains and aches, relax her mind and let her finish the practice by being rejuvenated, having enhanced her mobility, but also tone up her body and work out on her weight loss if this is what she is aiming at.

The importance and benefits though are not solely for the mother. Practicing in baby's presence creates positive energies with which baby can learn taking care of self, practicing strengthens the body, pranayama relaxes and connects body and mind, and place the seeds to a healthy lifestyle for its adulthood.

Practising Asanas

Although the following list of asanas with the given variations and modifications are considered to be safe to practice during pregnancy and after childbirth, it is advisable to have the healthcare provider's approval before doing so.

I personally encourage slow and steady movement on my Yoga practices and I would suggest when guiding your students, always consider possible mobility issues. Cardio type of exercise can be performed during pregnancy, but not in the way of up and down on the mat while practicing yoga. If you are guiding your prenatal class with any order from supine to standing and seated position, that might create discomfort, dizziness, increase in heart rate, but most importantly from my personal experience anxiety for having a personal yoga professional who does not understand my needs and ease on mobility up and down, especially as pregnancy progresses. It can be an agonizing time which is totally unnecessary if you value your personal and/ or professional relationship with your students. Decide your class plan in advance and plan the poses in a way that you will guide your class in one or two positions comfortably.

You may also consider having a back-up class planned! Yes! A pregnant woman may not be able to follow a full sitting class for example. Or if you have planned a supine position class she may experience dizziness and might want to exit the class. Or you may have planned asanas she is not into them that day or she doesn't feel comfortable performing those at that time. Be flexible, know your asanas and provide modifications whenever needed.

We, as qualified yoga teachers, specialized in pre-postnatal yoga we should have values such as patience, humility, compassion and commitment. Speaking of commitment, during her pregnancy, a woman may cancel many of the planned classes, and that may upset you as a yoga teacher because you depend on these classes financially. If she feels and knows you are there for her when she needs you most, you have many chances she will continue with you even after her baby is born for her postnatal practice. If she feels your frustration for not being able to attend a planned morning class maybe because of her possible morning sickness, she may also feel abandoned and that may harm her emotionally. Her hormones can be triggered by so many internal and external factors and your flexibility and commitment to her is really important. We are all in this niche to support and guide a healthy pregnancy but most importantly to welcome a healthy baby in life.

Thinking of safe practicing, always keep this mantra for your prenatal classes:

First Trimester: On all seated or standing asanas, keep the distance between the legs maximum to the width of the yoga mat.

Second Trimester: On all seated or standing asanas, keep the distance between the legs minimum to the edges of the mat. From second trimester onwards, always perform standing or balancing asanas with the support of a wall or a chair.

Third Trimester: On all seated or standing asanas, keep the legs as wide open as it feels comfortable and outside of the mat.

Asanas to avoid

Sun Salutations can even be a complete class, which requires a lot of physic which can lead to exhaustion at this phase of a woman's life. The modified Surya Namaskar can be practiced, however if while practicing, fatigue or dizziness or pain is felt should discontinue practice at once.

Locust Pose can add pressure to abdomen area and is advisable to avoid any similar asanas, as these might harm pregnancy and baby.

Naukasana can add pressure on abdomen and abdominal muscles which can stress the womb. Any similar asanas is advisable to be avoided during pregnancy.

Halasana can add pressure on core area which can affect pregnancy and baby's well development inside the womb.

First Trimester

First trimester can be challenging for many women, as in their physical level they will need to cope with nausea and morning sickness, fatigue and drowsiness.

To help the pregnancy get established, we need to always keep reminding that there should be no jerky movement in any part of the body, especially in the abdomen area. The movement should not have a compression effect in any part of the abdomen area. When practicing at this first trimester, our intention is not to achieve flexibility, but build strength to the body. Practitioner should go until the point there is no strain, and not to achieve the final position, whether this is a bend or a twist or a balancing pose. Objective for any practice is to stretch the regions we work with, without any overstretch. At any time, do not hold the breath. Only getting to the position is with breath awareness – like inhaling to raise hands up, and when on the final position breathing should be normal and continuous.

- Cat and Cow Stretch Pose – Marjariasana

- Child's Pose – Shashankasana

- Cow's Face Pose – Gomukhasana

- Head to Knee Pose – Janu Sirshasana

- Meditation Asanas

- One-Legged Prayer or Tree Pose – Eka Pada Pranamasana

- Pawanmuktasana Part 1

- Seated Cat & Cow Pose – Marjariasana

- Seated Twist or Marichi Pose – Marichyasana

- Standing Spinal Twist Pose – Katichakrasana

- Sun Salutation – Surya Namaskar (First Trimester)

- Swaying Palm Tree Pose – Tiryak Tadasana

- Triangle Pose – Trikonasana

- Vajrasana Group of Asanas

- Warrior I – Virabhadrasana I

- Warrior II – Virabhadrasana II

- Warrior III – Virabhadrasana II

Second Trimester

It is recommended to sit on Sukhasana while practicing any seated asanas during the prenatal period. From second trimester onwards the heel should not touch the belly and should create some space between the heel, perineum and belly to sit comfortably.

The following asanas can be considered as seated warm up or cooling down practices, which can also be given as a complete class. During the second trimester we recommend a lot of stretching, chest opening practices and gentle twists, which all will improve circulatory movement to prevent fluid retention on the third trimester. The would-be-mums usually feel and are on their maximum energy levels at that trimester and they usually ask for more than that, however, caution is our most objective. Pregnancy is not the time to practice strenuously as any practices will cause more fatigue. Instead, stretching will loosen muscles' tension, strengthen the muscles, encourage circulation to avoid fluid retention, and prepare the muscles for labor. By stretching, we also help our body to remove toxins and help the body to enter the third trimester in better shape and health. Twists will also help stretch the spine and the lower back as well as tone the spinal nerves.

Diaphragm, the respiratory muscle, is located just where the rib cage ends. As the pregnancy progresses towards the third trimester, the growing baby comes and squeezes and at times hits the diaphragm. This natural growth creates a lot of breathlessness for the would-be-mum. She will feel low or no energetic and with nearly no stamina at all in the body. In order to address these conditions, we do chest opening asanas and stretching to create space between the diaphragm and the belly. It is vital to practice these asanas to prepare the body for the third trimester, when the belly will naturally grow bigger, and the diaphragm will need the room to properly function up and down during inhalation and exhalation. Therefore, chest opening asanas will not only help respiratory system and oxygen flow for the would-be-mum, but also for her baby as well who still depends on mother's oxygen for healthy development.

As mentioned earlier in this book, it is advisable not to mix the trimesters on group classes. If this is not feasible, as a yoga teacher, you may not be able to go slow. In such cases, you have to have modifications in place or even alternate asanas. In order to achieve less energy loss during practicing, you may offer longer breaks between asanas and combine more pranayama techniques. You may also open your group class with a statement similar to *"Observe your body, listen to your body and your energy level. If something doesn't feel right, do not push yourself. Return to the original position and breathe"*.

- Bird Dog or Balancing Table Top Pose – Parsva Balasana

- Camel Pose – Ushtrasana

- Cat and Cow Stretch Pose – Marjariasana

- Chair Pose – Utkatasana

- Child's Pose – Shashankasana

- Cow's Face Pose – Gomukhasana

- Donkey Kicks Straight Raised Leg

- Gate Pose – Parighasana

- Goddess Pose – Kaliasana

- Head to Knee Pose – Janu Sirshasana

- Kneeling Asanas

- Lion Pose – Simhasana

- One-Legged King Pigeon Pose – Eka Pada Rajakapotasana

- Roaring Lion Pose – Simhagarjanasana

- Seated Camel Pose – Ushtrasana in Sukhasana

- Seated Cat & Cow Pose – Marjariasana

- Seated Eagle Pose – Garudasana

- Seated Palm Tree Pose – Parvatasana in Sukhasana

- Seated Prayer Flow – Sukhasana Namaste Hands Vinyasa

- Seated Side Bend – Parsva Sukhasana

- Seated Spinal Twist – Parivritti in Sukhasana

- Seated Twist or Marichi Pose – Marichyasana

- Spiraled Head to Knee Pose – Parivritti Janu Sirshasana

- Sun Salutation – Surya Namaskar (Second & Third Trimester)

- Thread the Needle Flow – Urdhva Mukha Pasasana Vinyasa

- Vajrasana Group of Asanas

- Wide Angled Seated Forward Bend – Upavistha Konasana

Third Trimester

The main difference between the asanas given on second and third trimester, lies mostly on the full squatting practices given on late pregnancy. Further, most women find it challenging to practice most asanas because of the growing belly. Third trimester should be treated as a restorative yoga, taking the extra time to come in and out from each position.

This trimester comes with a lot of fluid retention in upper and lower body. To make sure there is not so much fluid trapped in the body, it is required to do a lot of stretching. Half and full squatting is necessary to help pelvis open up, and especially as the would-be-mum enters the labor time. Practicing with any support system is vital, even if the practitioner is experienced. A wall should be used for standing asanas to maintain balance and stability as the body gravity is changed with the extra weight and the growing belly. A cushion when necessary is vital to avoid compression of the belly or general overstretching.

- Bird Dog or Balancing Table Top Pose – Parsva Balasana

- Bridge or Shoulder Pose – Kandharasana or Setu Bandha Sarvangasana

- Cat and Cow Stretch Pose – Marjariasana

- Child's Pose – Shashankasana

- Cow's Face Pose – Gomukhasana

- Duck Walking – Karandavasana

- Goddess Pose – Kaliasana

- Half Forward Bend – Ardha Uttanasana

- Head to Knee Pose – Janu Sirshasana

- One-Legged Prayer or Tree Pose – Eka Pada Pranamasana

- Seated Camel Pose – Ushtrasana in Sukhasana

- Seated Cat & Cow Pose – Marjariasana

- Seated Eagle Pose – Garudasana

- Seated Palm Tree Pose – Parvatasana in Sukhasana

- Seated Prayer Flow – Sukhasana Namaste Hands Vinyasa

- Seated Side Bend – Parsva Sukhasana

- Seated Spinal Twist – Parivritti in Sukhasana

- Seated Twist or Marichi Pose – Marichyasana

- Squatting Asanas

- Sun Salutation – Surya Namaskar (Second & Third Trimester)

- Swaying Palm Tree Pose – Tiryak Tadasana

- Vajrasana Group of Asanas

- Wide Angled Seated Forward Bend – Upavistha Konasana

Fourth Trimester

What a wonderful journey! It may have had some discomfort, it may still have, but look at your baby!

Hold it, hug it, kiss it, care for it, love it!

The body will be in ache for some time, but Yoga With Me is your partner to that journey! When practicing during pregnancy, you are practicing for you and your baby. When you are practicing post childbirth, your main focus is to feel energetic, rejuvenated, calm and also release body tension arising mainly from bad body posture, fatigue and sometimes malnutrition. Never forget yourself! You are just the two of you and you deserve to relax, be active, be you the way it makes you happy! Free time may seem limited while nursing the baby, may even seem this is the only thing you do! Enjoy this time of loving care and dependence, and remember that babies grow rapidly! This phase will soon be a nice memory!

Even from day 1 post childbirth, you may practice the Pawanmuktasana 1, called the Anti-Rheumatic Group, which help the physical movement of bones, joints, ligaments and muscles to relieve from pain and tension. When the physical body has recovered from childbirth, practice can consume. However, always remember that the body and organs need time to return to its normal shape and positioning, and for at least the first 6 months' post childbirth practice should be with cautiousness and awareness in order to avoid any injuries or tearing of the muscles.

Yoga for Breastfeeding

Practicing yoga even while breastfeeding, is not only great for the mum but also for the baby being exposed to yoga practices. For example, if nursing lying on the side, variations of Anantasana can be performed even during feeding. Whereas, Gomukhasana and any arms and shoulders movements can relieve tension from the upper body and improve body posture. Practicing Surya Namaskar (Second & Third Trimester) can further connect body and mind, strengthen the body and help with post-pregnancy weight loss. Standing asanas while holding the baby can increase stamina and strengthen the body, and inverted asanas will improve the metabolism.

The following asanas improve blood circulation and aid the secretion of prolactin and milk from the mammary glands for the period a mother feeds her baby:

- Back Stretching Pose – Paschimottanasana

- Bridge or Shoulder Pose – Kandharasana or Setu Bandha Sarvangasana

- Camel Pose – Ushtrasana

- Cat and Cow Stretch Pose – Marjariasana

- Child's Pose – Shashankasana

- Cobra Pose – Bhujangasana

- Cow's Face Pose – Gomukhasana

- Dog Pose – Shvanasana

- Donkey Kicks Straight Raised Leg

- Elbow Rotation – Kehuni Chakra

- Equestrian Pose – Ashwa Sanchalanasana

- Extended Puppy Pose – Uttana Shishosana

- Flapping Fish Pose – Matsya Kridasana

- Half Butterfly – Ardha Titali

- Half Camel Pose – Ardha Ushtrasana

- Half Forward Bend – Ardha Uttanasana

- Half Moon Pose – Ardha Chandrasana

- Head to Knee Pose – Janu Sirshasana

- Leg Lock Pose – Supta Pawanmuktasana

- Mountain Pose – Parvatasana

- Raised Arms Pose – Hasta Utthanasana

- Seated Camel Pose – Ushtrasana in Sukhasana

- Seated Cat & Cow Pose – Marjariasana

- Seated Palm Tree Pose – Parvatasana in Sukhasana

- Seated Side Bend – Parsva Sukhasana

- Seated Spinal Twist – Parivritti in Sukhasana

- Shoulder Socket Rotation – Skandha Chakra

- Side-Reclining Leg Lift Pose – Anantasana

- Spiraled Head to Knee Pose – Parivritti Janu Sirshasana

- Standing Spinal Twist Pose – Katichakrasana

- Universal Spinal Twist – Shava Udarakarshanasana

- Vajrasana Group of Asanas

- Wind Releasing Pose – Vayu Nishkasana

Yoga for Non-Breastfeeding

Physically, the same applies to all mums whether they still breastfeed their baby or not. When breastfeeding is ended, the woman should be still focusing on poses that will support her upper body, especially in the back, shoulders and neck area. The selected asanas will support the body in firming and toning up the core, and maintaining overall strength. For the mum who nurses with the bottle, she is not in lactation, and has fully recovered from childbirth, all asanas are allowed and she can be treated as a normal practitioner.

The same list of asanas given to breastfeeding mums as well as the following can be practiced:

- Bird Dog or Balancing Table Top Pose – Parsva Balasana

- Corpse Pose – Shavasana

- Cow's Face Pose – Gomukhasana

- Extended Triangle Pose – Utthita Trikonasana

- Full Butterfly – Poorna Titali Asana

- Half Lotus Pose – Ardha Padmasana

- Hero's Meditation Pose – Dhyana Veerasana

- Leg Rotation – Padachakrasana

- Pulling the Rope – Rajju Karshanasana

- Raised Leg Pose – Padotthanasana

- Swaying Palm Tree Pose – Tiryak Tadasana

Yoga with the Baby

This chapter is for Motherhood Yoga and its first year, where the woman has fully recovered from childbirth, the baby is not sleeping and active, and it is time to practice yoga, but how? During yoga practice with the baby, relaxation and pranayama may be impossible – unless the baby is sleeping, is quite or not crawling, where it would be like a common yoga practice. If you are having around a crawling baby, that means that your student is way after her 6th or 7th month post-delivery, which commonly places practice as safe. If the practitioner had a C-section, it is always recommended to have healthcare advisor's approval before following the list of asanas presented on this chapter.

If you are a mother yourself, or if you have been observing another woman during her post-delivery period you have noticed that there might be many days that practicing yoga amongst other things may be challenging. What needs to be remembered is that during this period which lasts from Day 1 to anywhere up to 5 years, self-practicing or practicing with a coach in the presence of the baby and later child can be fun, interactive and creative. If any of the two or more participants (usually applies for mother and children) feel at any point frustration, the practice itself loses the amazing vibes of calmness and mindfulness. The fun time is until baby starts crawling! Yes! Babies until they start crawling, usually they sit and stay where you position them, and is easier to manage the practice in time and in selection of the sequence. While practicing with the baby, the sequence will not be rich in variety, however it can never be boring, as it is in full interaction with the baby, and is also getting more advanced with baby's weight and height growth. Many asanas can be practiced with the baby, depending on its age and mood! Standing asanas while holding the baby can help tone up the body and inverted asanas will improve metabolism. Seated asanas whilst reading a book or playing, supine and prone asanas, arms and legs movements, can also be practiced with the baby. What you need to do is be creative!

For those women returning to work, this period may create mixed feelings of happiness of getting out of the house or guilt having to leave the baby with someone else! It is all on perception, and other than asanas that can offer quality time and bonding when co-practicing with the baby, it is also important to self-practice Yoga Nidra, pranayama, om chanting and meditation to help balance the emotions. The combination of two or more yogic practices will definitely help to come to a relaxed state for both mind and body. Motherhood after all, is all about awareness, self-control, patience, care, unconditional love and understanding!

On my pranayama practices, I was co-practicing with my son the Bhramari for its great benefits for me and him when he started mimicking me! I keep co-practicing with both my kids the Shanmukhi Mudra, because it can be used as Peekaboo game for them and at the same time offer me some moments of mental relaxation! The baby and later toddler is having fun with these practices and stays energetic either by crawling or running to hide somewhere and the mother takes a few moments to herself to complete 1 round. However, if the practitioner is suffering from postpartum depression should not practice Shanmukhi Mudra.

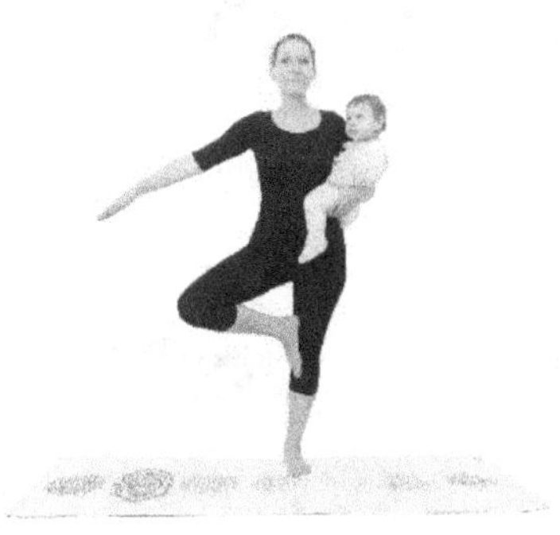

Eka Pada Pranamasana

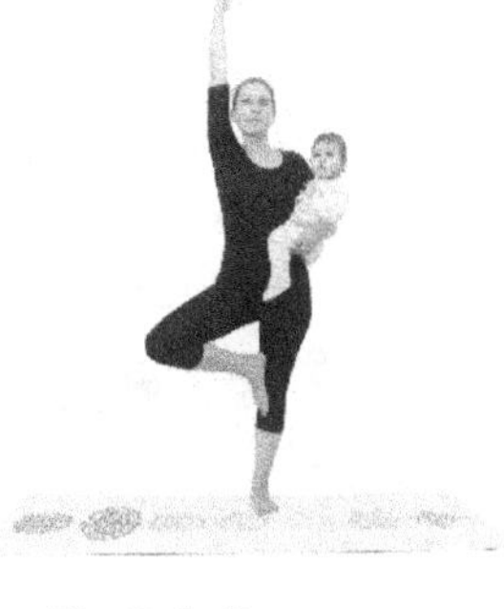

Eka Pada Pranamasana

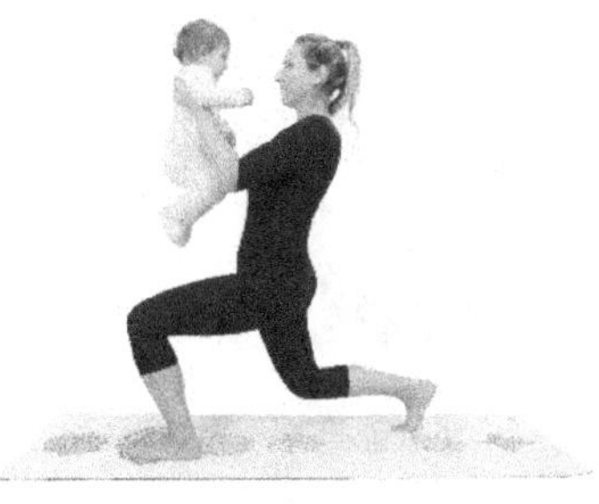

Ashwa Sanchalanasana

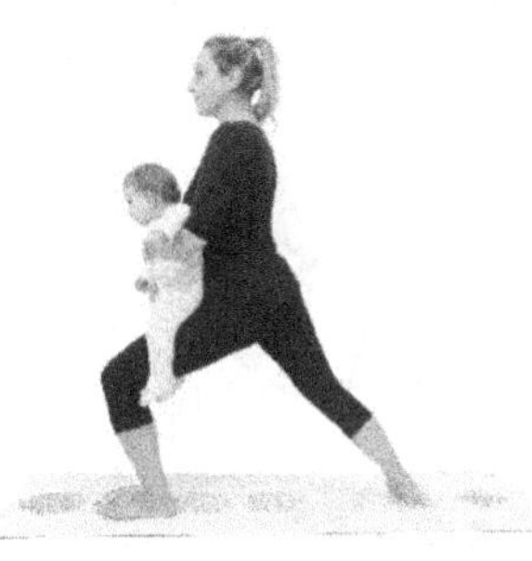

Virabhadrasana II

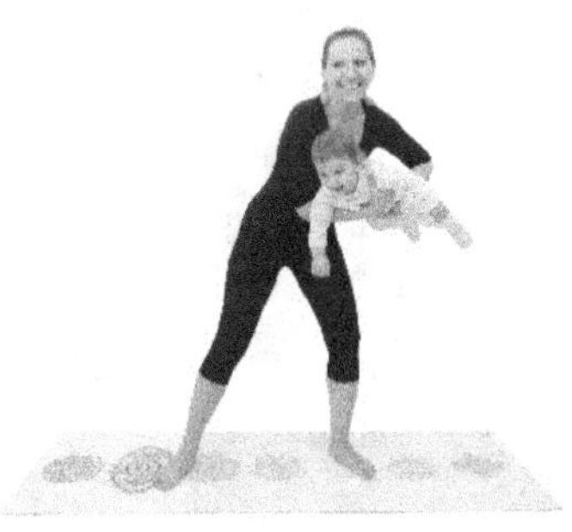

Katichakrasana

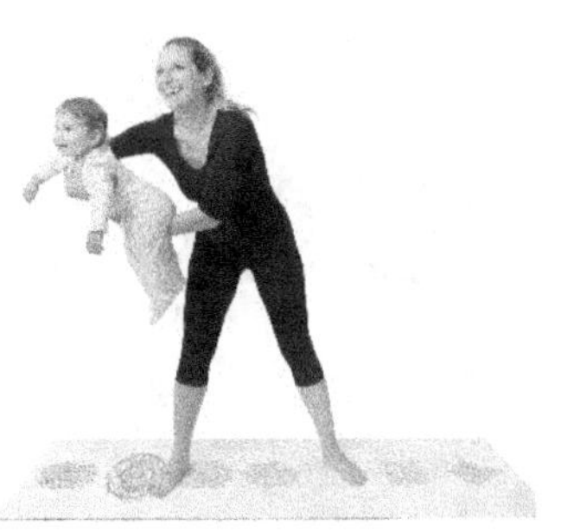

Katichakrasana

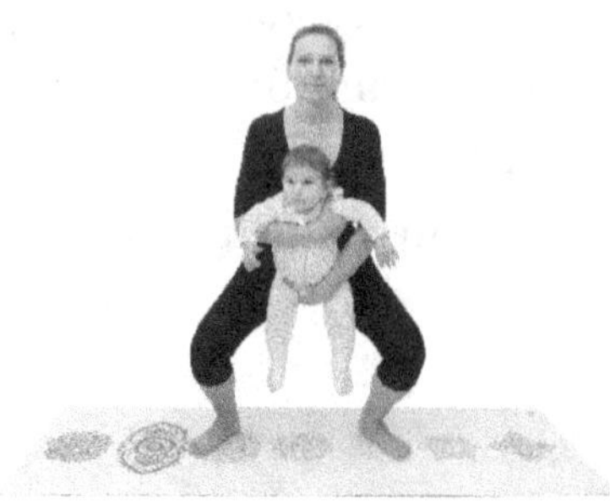

Kaliasana

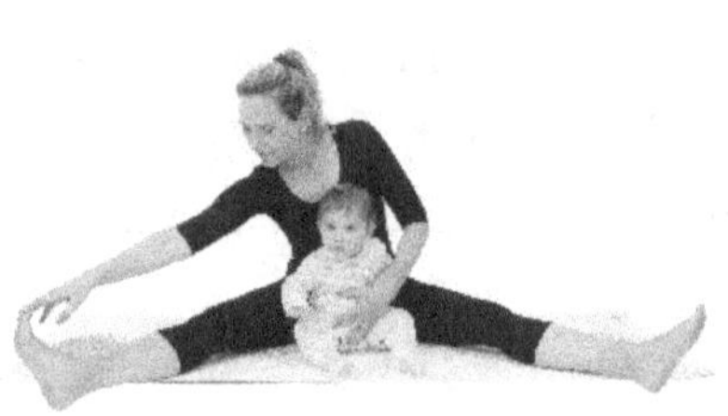

Upavistha Konasana

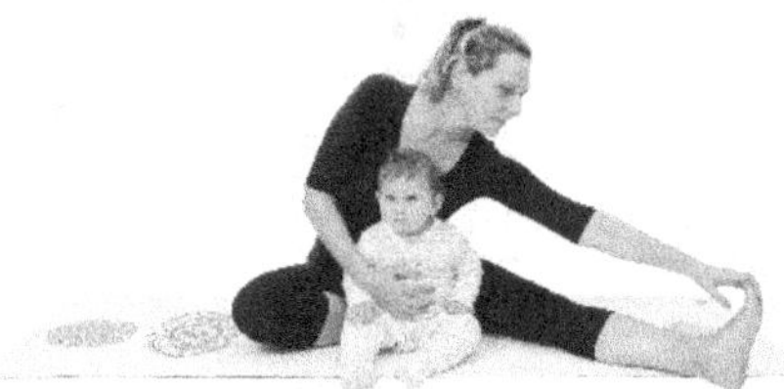

Janu Sirshasana

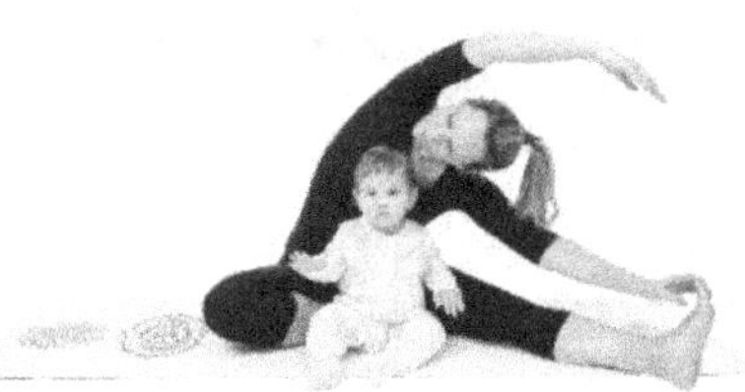

Parivritti Janu Sirshasana

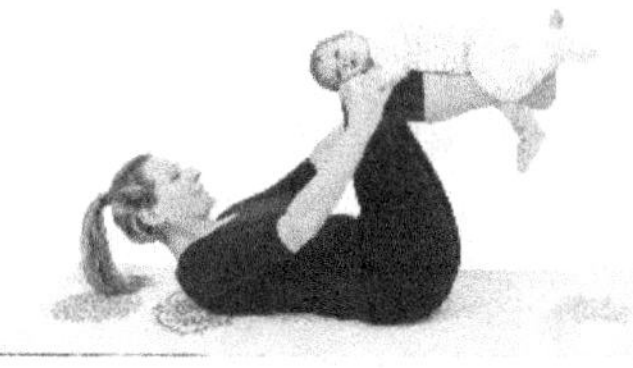

Supta Pawanmuktasana

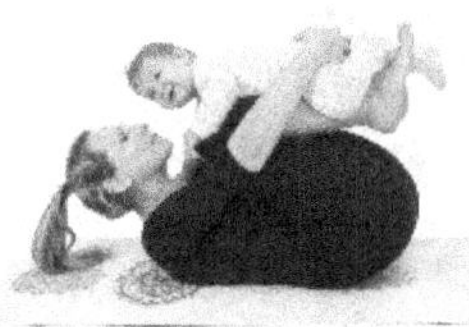

Supta Pawanmuktasana

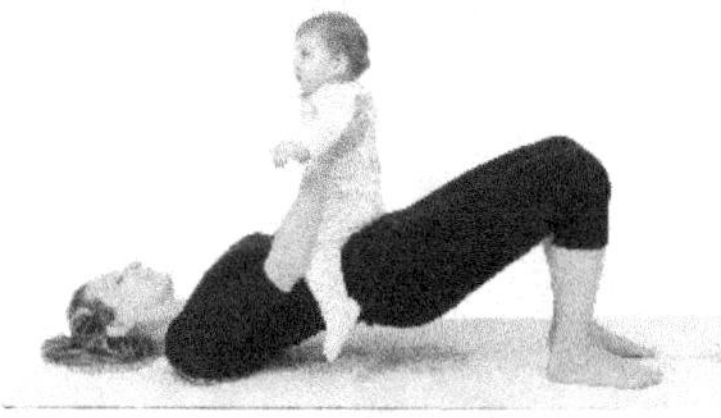

Kandharasana

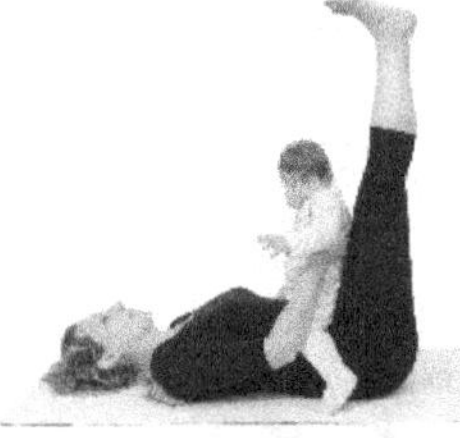

Padotthanasana 90° angle

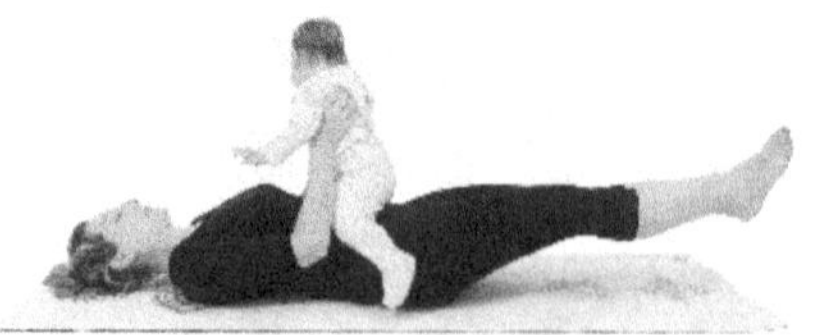

Padotthanasana 30° angle

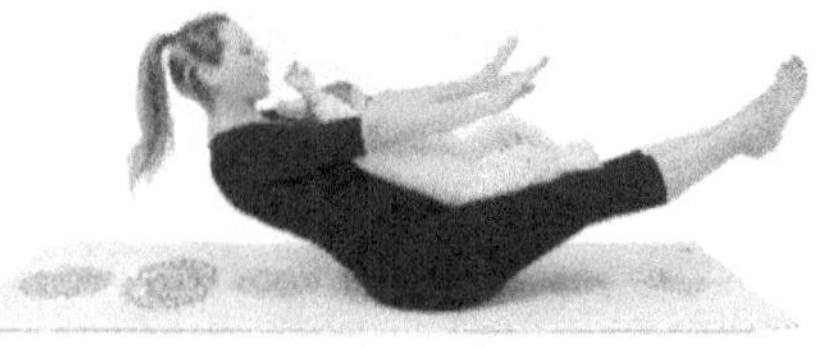

Naukasana

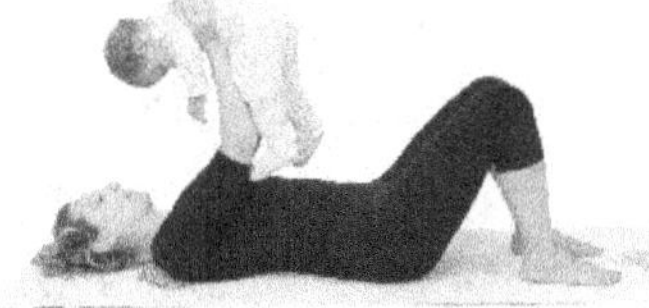

Supine Arms Strenthening Up

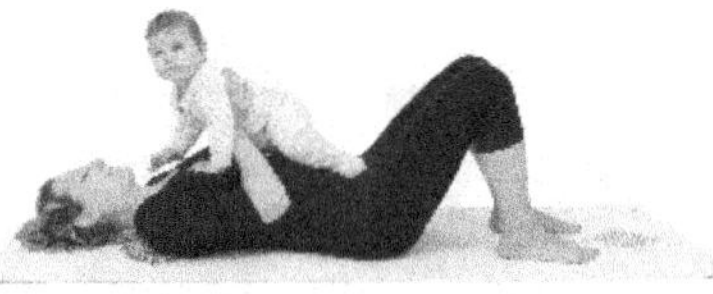

Supine Arms Strenthening Down

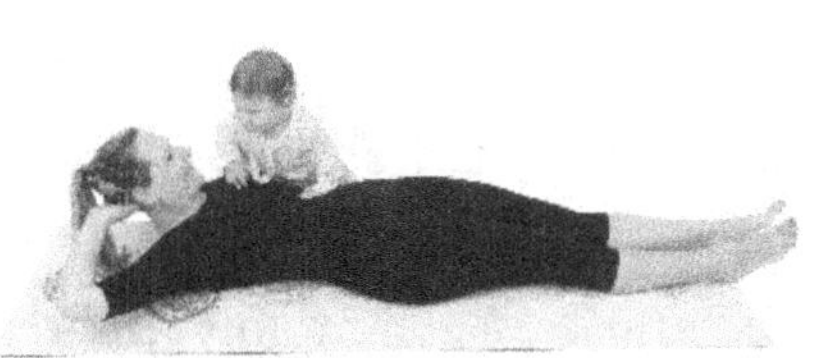

Crunches

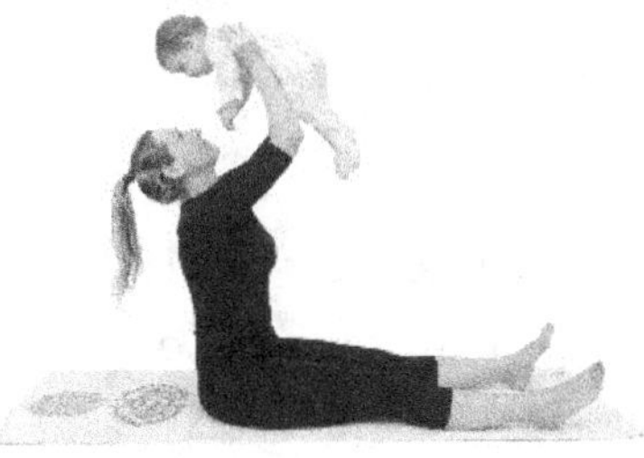

Seated Arms Strenthening Up

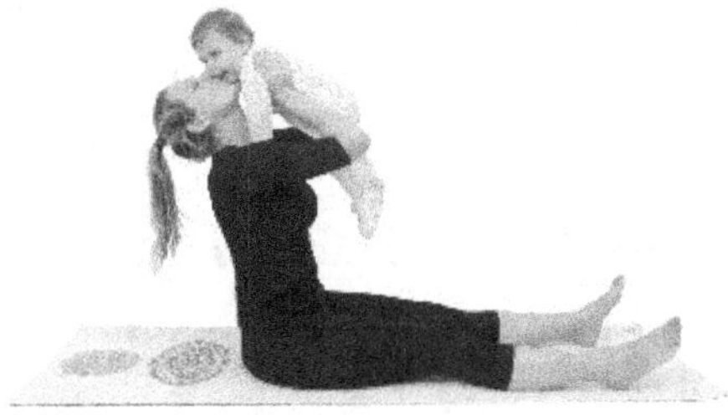

Seated Arms Strenthening Down

Kegel Exercises

Kegel exercises are implicitly connected to the pelvic region and muscles. Can be practiced anytime and anywhere and they are essential to women of all ages and stages of life, as these increase control over the bladder, and strengthen the pelvic floor which supports the vagina, uterus and bowel. A strong pelvic floor may help the second stage of labor to be shorter, and post childbirth may also help recover the area.

Practice: These are practices that cannot be shown, but felt. Correct way of practicing is to locate and squeeze the pelvic floor muscles without engaging the abdomen, buttock or leg muscles. Practice makes perfect anything! These can be quick exercises where the muscles are rapidly tightened and then relaxed; or slow exercises when the muscles are tightened for 10 seconds and then relaxed. Kegels are more efficient when each squeeze is as tight as possible. Can practice 10 rapid and 10 slow squeezes, 4-5 times a day, in any position, i.e. seated, standing, supine position.

Method 1: By identifying the pelvic muscles around the bladder opening, start and stop the urine stream. If able to stop mid-stream, then the pelvic floor muscles are used.

Method 2: Tighten the pelvic muscles around the back passage. The feeling should be as holding back wind.

Method 3: Engage the pelvic floor muscles upwards.

Benefits: Kegel exercises create flexibility and tone up all the pelvic floor muscles and help on constipation. Frequent practitioners it is unlikely to have hemorrhoids during pregnancy.

Precautions: If a woman is suffering from vaginal or pelvic pain should consult her healthcare advisor before practicing. If there is cervical stitching should not practice until recovery.

Pawanmuktasana Part 1

The warm-up and cooling down is as important as the actual practice of asanas itself. A warm-up can be performed even during pregnancy or in therapeutic yoga, and can also be practiced as a full session itself at any point of someone's life, in which occasion, the counts and rounds should be increased for the practice to be more effective.

On the physical level, these practices release toxins accumulated in body joints therefore can help prevention of rheumatics and arthritics and osteoporosis on the body. Especially after childbirth, a woman can attract arthritis, low bone density, osteoporosis or any disease related to the bones and joints. In all human joints there is a fluid called *synovial fluid* which works like a lubricating gel for the joints to be nicely movable. When we move our joints in a proper direction, the health and quantity of synovial fluid remains intact in the body and as we grow or as a woman reaches menopause, at that time is unlikely for a person to have joints' health issues. These practices are all extremely beneficial for numbness and tingling effects as they keep the bones, blood vessels, ligaments, tendons, fascia, nerves, muscles and joints in a proper shape and toned up. The minerals within the body, such as uric acid deposits are lowered and body feels lighter.

On the spiritual level, these practices are important because not only they remove energy blockages, but also, if we think of Ayurveda, these ease the Vata Dosha, the wind element accumulated in the joints responsible for the movement and energy in our bodies. On a certain level, these practices help remove the pranic blockages which help prana, the breath and the oxygen within the body to flow correctly. As prana is connected to the breath, breath is connected to the nervous system, parasympathetic and sympathetic, Ida and Pingala energies, so on a pranic level, when this flows without any blockages a person can have a better mind and body connection.

If we talk about anatomy during a pregnancy, major systems get impacted, especially the Circulatory System, Nervous System, Respiratory System,

Digestive System and the Endocrine System. These practices really help to bring systems back in order and especially if practiced daily, at the same time for a week or two, a person can experience drastic increase on energy levels. The following practices are really important during pregnancy because all the fluid retention can be taken care of and the circulatory system is generally helped to perform better. These can be performed even at the very late stage of pregnancy or even when labor has started, with great results to divert mind from pain and manage the labor pain. Especially for the post-delivery recovery, these practices are extremely beneficial to help body get back to its known condition and prevent fluid retention and all the above mentioned.

During the warm-up and cooling down, usually there is no need for periodic rest, as the sequence followed is to help the muscles warm up and cool down accordingly, release any tension from the joints, increase the awareness on every part of the body, helping at the same time the mind to relax from any thoughts. Mind is focused on mentally counting the repetitions to complete each round, therefore any uninvited thoughts are eliminated and concentration and balance between mind and body is achieved during practicing Yoga.

Note:

If practicing these asanas as a warm-up or cooling down, maximum 5-8 counts are sufficient.

If using this list of asanas for a full class, 2 or 3 rounds of 10-20 counts are sufficient; the number of rounds always depends upon your class time, planning and body parts you want to work out, but most importantly body's capacity.

There is no need for someone to do all the stages or variations of an asana; simply select and plan your class accordingly. If using these asanas as a full class and for example you have been warming-up Neck Left-to-Right Movements, then on cooling down you may consider giving the Neck Rotation Movement or any other neck variation.

Leg Movements

All these practices are for the lower limbs and are extremely beneficial as they help in blood circulation and release of any tension on muscles and joints. In particular, knee and ankle joints and muscles hold a lot of tension as they support the weight and movement of the whole body, therefore lower limbs are relieved from tiredness and cramps and help prevent edema, spider veins, fluid retention, venous thrombosis.

1. Base Position – Prarambhik Sthiti

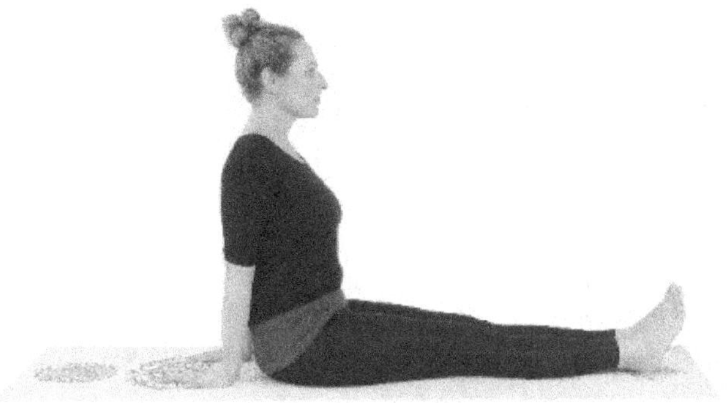

Practice: Sit with the legs outstretched, and if on:

First Trimester: Feet close together but not touching

Second Trimester: Feet apart, open to the width of the yoga mat.

Third Trimester: Feet wider apart.

Place the palms of the hands behind the buttocks and slightly lean back by using the arms to support the back. Can have a cushion or back support to help body to lean back if hands behind the buttocks are not comfortable. The elbows, back, spine, neck and head to be comfortably straight. Sense what feels more comfortable and accordingly position body taking under consideration the feet distance according to pregnancy trimester. *If practicing this pose for relaxation purposes, can maintain position for 2-3 minutes with eyes closed.*

2. Toe Bending – Padanguli Naman

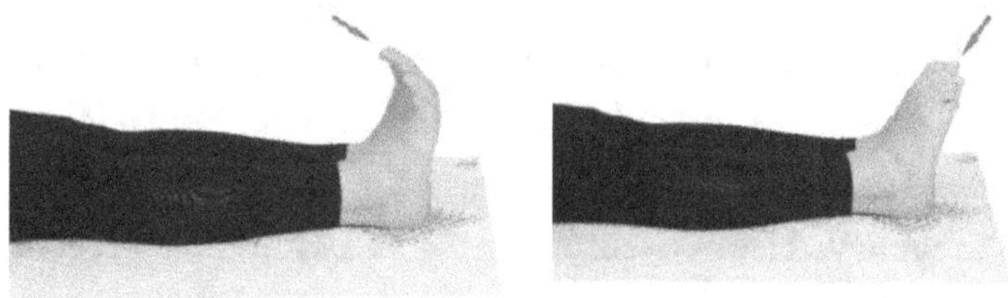

Practice: While on Base Position, move only the toes of both feet slowly to contract them and flex them for 8 counts; hold each move for a few seconds. The feet should be upright and the ankles relaxed.

Breathing: Inhale to contract and squeeze toes. Exhale to flex and spread toes out.

Awareness: On toes stretching and breathing.

3. Ankle Bending – Goolf Naman

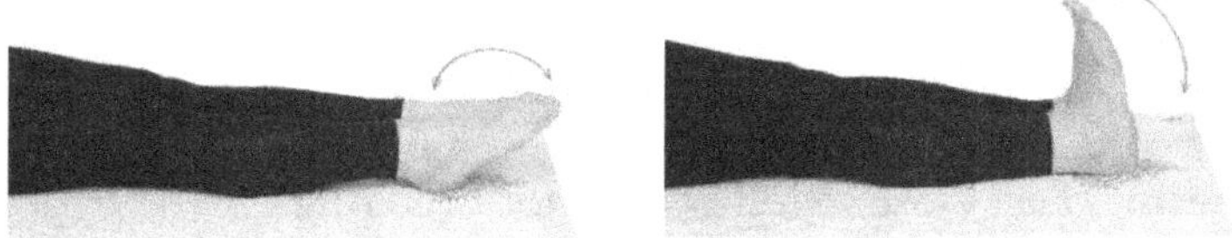

Practice: While on Base Position, stretch feet by bending them forward, trying to touch the floor. On that move should feel stretch around the shin bone and quadriceps area. Bending should be from the ankle joints. Hold each move for a few seconds.

Variation 1: Practice with alternate feet; 5-8 counts on each foot.

Variation 2: Practice both feet together; 5-8 counts total.

Breathing: Inhale to move feet backward and towards the body; Exhale to stretch feet forward to touch the floor.

Awareness: On the stretch of the foot, ankle, calf, leg and breathing.

4. Ankle Rotation – Goolf Chakra

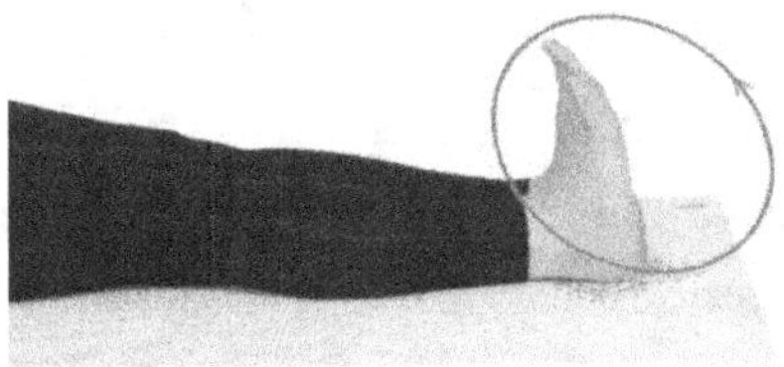

Practice: While on Base Position, heels should be kept on the ground during the practice and feet should be separated to ease practice. Rotation to be performed in to a full 360° circle.

Variation 1: Rotate right foot 5-8 counts clockwise and anticlockwise. Repeat with left foot.

Variation 2: Rotate both feet together 5-8 counts in the same direction clockwise and anticlockwise.

Breathing: Inhale to rotate feet up. Exhale to rotate feet down.

Awareness: On breathing and feet rotation from the ankles.

5. Knee Bending – Janu Naman

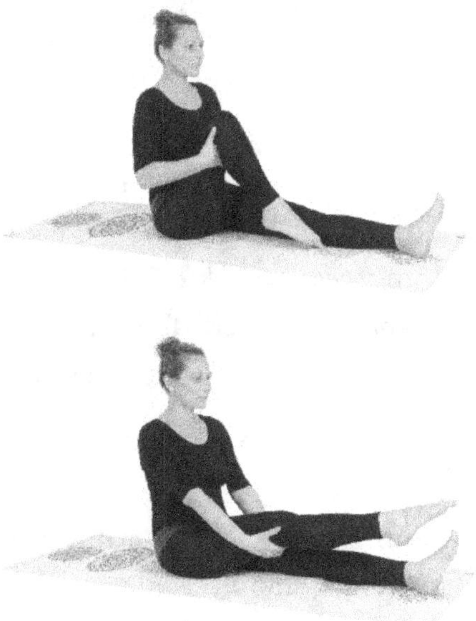

Practice: While on Base Position, keep the head and spine straight, bend the right knee and grasp the right thigh or kneecap with the hands. On the bent move, the leg should open diagonally so the inner thigh of bent leg – groin area should not hit the belly. Leg may not come close to the body; it is fine to be slightly extended. Try to keep the bent leg's heel to a parallel level with the left knee. Straighten right leg by pulling up the kneecap by straightening the right arm. Keep the right heel as high or low to the ground as it feels comfortable and safe. Practice for 5-8 counts and repeat the same with the left leg.

Breathing: Inhale while straightening leg. Exhale while bending leg.

Awareness: On breathing and movement so thigh doesn't hit belly.

6. Half Butterfly – Ardha Titali

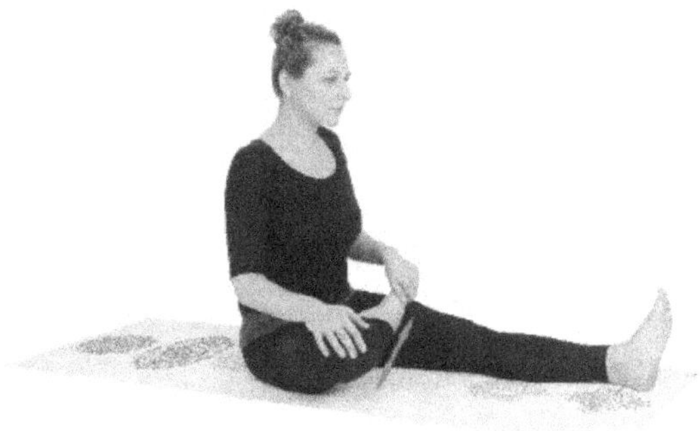

Practice: While on Base Position, keep the head and spine straight, trunk to be stable. Use cushions or yoga blocks below the knees and hips area for support, so there is no unnecessary jerk on the pelvic and abdomen area. Place right foot comfortably on the left thigh. Place right hand on top of bent right knee. Hold right foot toes with left hand.

Second & Third Trimester:

Place your heel away from perinea area, at a distance where right heel is facing the left knee. The left leg should be diagonally open and positioned outside of the yoga mat. The right ankle should be comfortably resting on the floor in front of the perineum at approximately 1-foot distance or 30 centimeters or 12 inch. Slowly move upward and downward the right knee.

Variation 1: Breath Synchronization (slow movement)

Inhale and gently move the right knee up. Exhale and push the knee down and without any force. Practice slowly for 8 counts up and down. Repeat the same with the left leg.

Variation 2: Without Breath Synchronization (fast movement)

Do not strain; let the knee spring up by itself. Practice continuously and at a faster speed for 20 or 30 counts up and down. Breathing should be normal and not related to the movement of the knee. Repeat the same with the left leg.

Awareness: For Variation 1, on breathing, while relaxing the inner thigh muscles and focusing on the knee, ankle and hip joints movement. For Variation 2, on the knee movement. For both Variations, one should be cautious when the knee is coming up towards the body, not to hit the belly.

Benefits: This is an excellent asana to loosen up the knee and hip joints. Can be performed before meditative poses.

Counter Pose: Practice Janu Naman with fully outstretched the extended leg diagonally. Try to slowly bend and extend the leg in a slow and careful movement. That way will ensure knee joint is realigned correctly, especially if practicing more than 20 or 30 repetitions.

7. Full Butterfly – Poorna Titali Asana

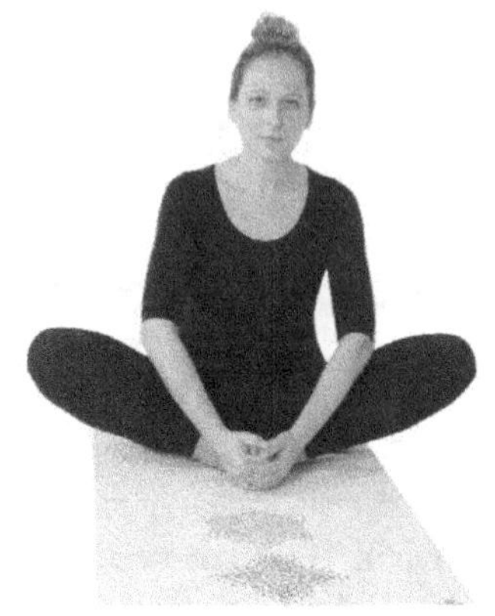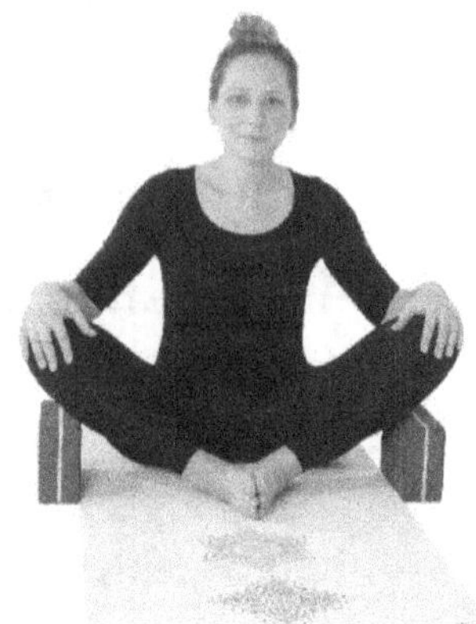

Practice: While on Base Position, keep the head and spine straight, trunk to be stable. Use cushions or yoga blocks below the knees and hips area for support, so there is no unnecessary jerk on the pelvic and abdomen area. Bend the knees, bring the soles of the feet together, keeping the heels as far as possible from the perineum as possible (approximately 1-foot distance or 30 centimeters or 12 inch). Adjust distance to comfort zone so belly can be nicely accommodated. Position your hands either on top of the knees, or grasp the knees, or grasp the toes, whichever feels more comfortable and slightly do the movement in a slow motion. The legs should move up maximum until the point the inner thighs are not hitting the belly. Try to bring the knees closer to the ground. Practice with a nice and smooth movement from the hip area for 30 counts.

Breathing: Inhale when rotating leg upwards. Exhale when rotating leg downward.

Awareness: Be more mindful of not hitting the belly part of the body.

Hand and Shoulder Movements

The hand and wrist asanas are important, as they can relieve stiffness and tension from the related joints caused by writing, typing, driving or heavy hand work. The shoulder asanas can be beneficial to the body as they maintain the shape of shoulders and chest, but also relieve aches from bad body posture, pressure in cervical spondylitis and frozen shoulder. They are extremely beneficial for numbness and tingling effects in the hands area which also have the tendency to accumulate a lot of fluid and toxins, which, when they are accumulated after the pregnancy may lead to arthritis or osteoporosis.

During the pregnancy and postnatal duration these are beneficial for breast tenderness or breast enlargement and chest soreness. If a woman feels breathless during her pregnancy, especially during the third trimester, these movements can get instant energy to her body. Furthermore, with awareness on slow breathing/movement fulfils the extra requirement of oxygen in the body.

When practicing, if at any point practitioner feels tired, can shake gently the hands for a few breaths and consume practice. Can be performed in either standing or any cross-legged seated position or seated in a chair.

8. Hand Clenching – Mushtika Bandhana

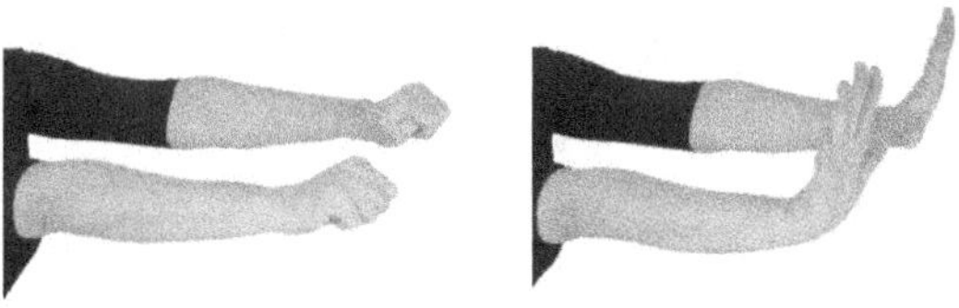

Practice: Extend hands in front of the body and make a fist with the thumb inside the fist. While inhaling clench a fist, while exhaling, extend the fingers wide open. Opening of the fist and extension of the fingers to be rapid and forceful to feel a nice stretch on the whole palm area from wrist to fingers.

Breathing: Inhale on clenching the fist. Exhale on fingers' extension.

Awareness: On breathing and palm of the hand movement.

9. Wrist Joint Rotation – Manibandha Chakra

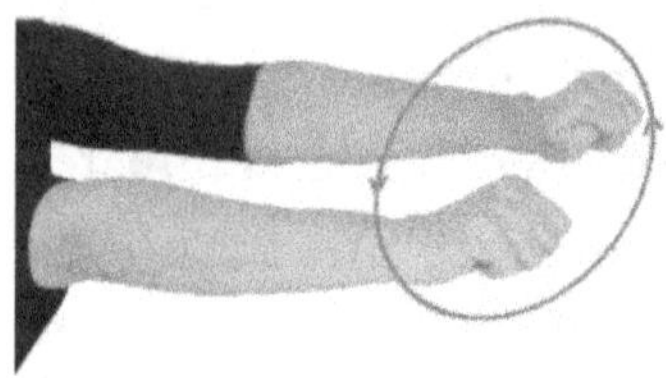

Practice: Extend hands in front of the body and make a fist with the thumb inside the fist. Make a full wrist rotation to one direction clockwise and anticlockwise for maximum awareness and synchronization of the breath.

Variation 1:

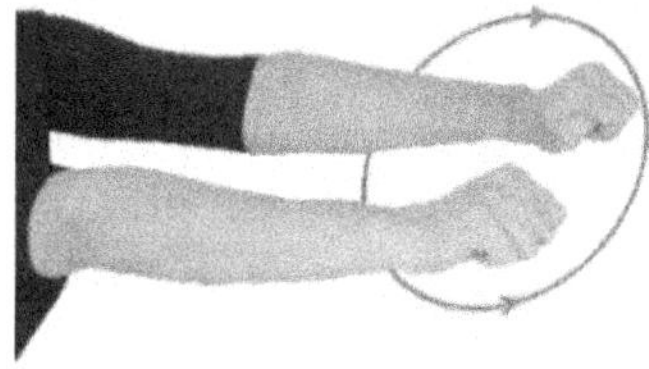

Can also practice rotation towards opposite directions by experienced practitioners; for beginners may become difficult and challenging for breath synchronization. The movement should be slow and steady so only the hands are moving and a nice stretch is experienced on both upper and lower arm.

Breathing: Inhale on upward rotation. Exhale on downward rotation.

Awareness: On breathing and gentle full rotation movement.

10. Wrist Bending – Manibandha Naman

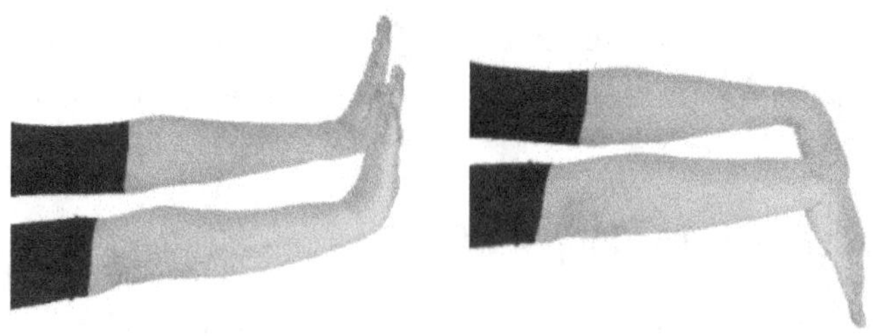

Practice: Extend hands in front of the body with fingers pointing the sky. With spine sitting straight, should stretch the hands to get the feeling as if pushing against a wall and feel the tension and stretch in the whole upper and lower arm.

Breathing: Inhale on extension of the wrist up. Exhale on flexion of the wrist down.

Awareness: On breathing and wrist movement to feel maximum stretch.

11. Elbow Bending – Kehuni Naman

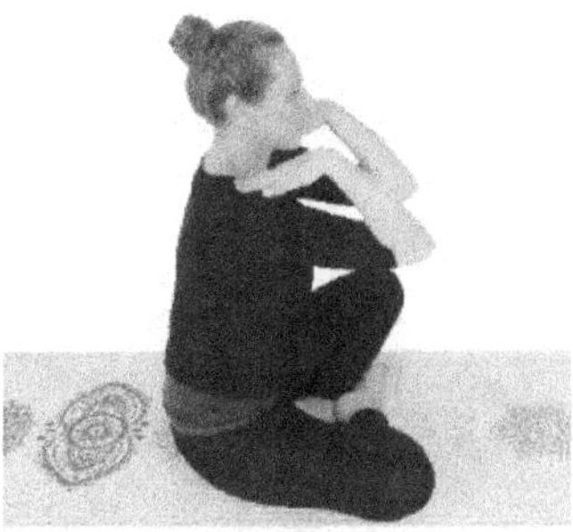

Practice: Bring the hands in front of the body, palms facing the sky. Inhale to straighten the arms, exhale to bend elbows and rest fingers on the shoulders. Upper arms should remain parallel to the ground. Repeat for 5-8 counts with normal and continuous breathing and movement.

Variation 1:

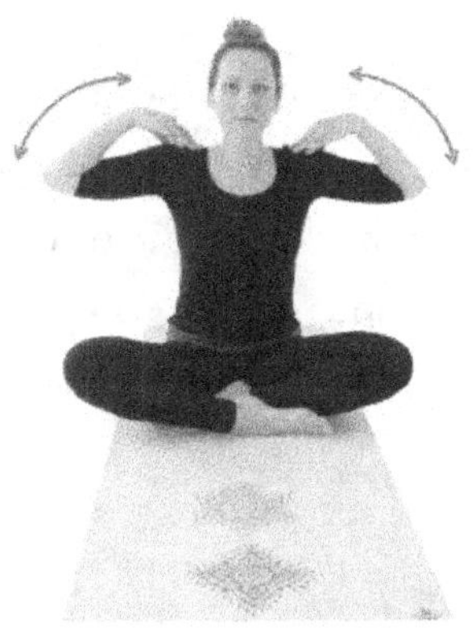

Extend the arms to the side at shoulders level, the hands open and palms facing the sky. Inhale to straighten the arms sideways, exhale to bend elbows and rest fingers on the shoulders. Upper arms should remain parallel to the ground. Repeat for 10 counts with continuous breathing and movement.

Breathing: Inhale on straightening the arms (in front of the body or sideways). Exhale on bending the arms.

Awareness: On breathing and the movement of the elbow joint and the arm muscles.

12. Shoulder Socket Rotation – Skandha Chakra

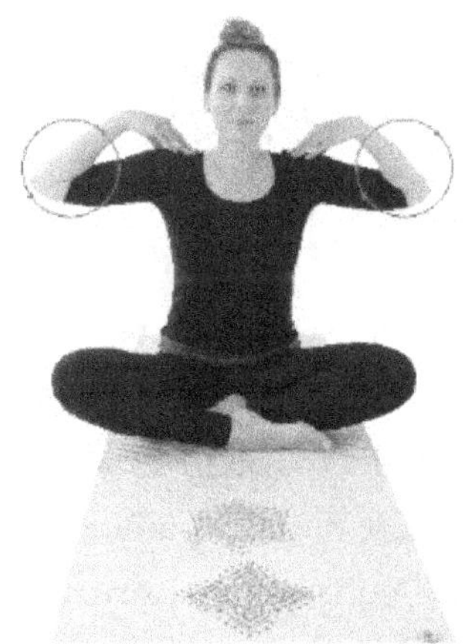

Practice: Touch with the left fingers the left shoulder, and keep the right hand on the right knee with the spine straight. Rotate the left elbow for a full circle. On the forward movement bring elbow in front of the chest. On the upward movement attempt to touch the left ear. On the backward movement stretch the left arm back. On the downward movement attempt to touch the left side of the trunk. Practice slowly 5-8 times clockwise and anticlockwise. Repeat the same with the right side.

Variation:

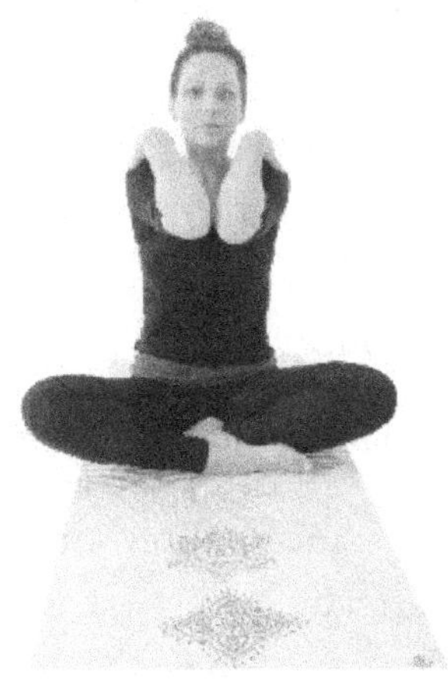

This is a chest opening asana. Touch with the right fingers the right shoulder, with the left fingers the left shoulder and rotate both elbows at the same time for a full circle. On the forward movement attempt to touch the elbows in front of the chest. On the upward movement attempt to touch the ears for chest stretching and opening. On the backward movement, stretch the arms back. On the downward movement attempt to touch the trunk sides. Practice slowly for 5-8 times clockwise and anticlockwise.

Breathing: Inhale on upward movement. Exhale on downward movement.

Awareness: On breathing and the shoulder stretch.

13. Elbow Rotation – Kehuni Chakra

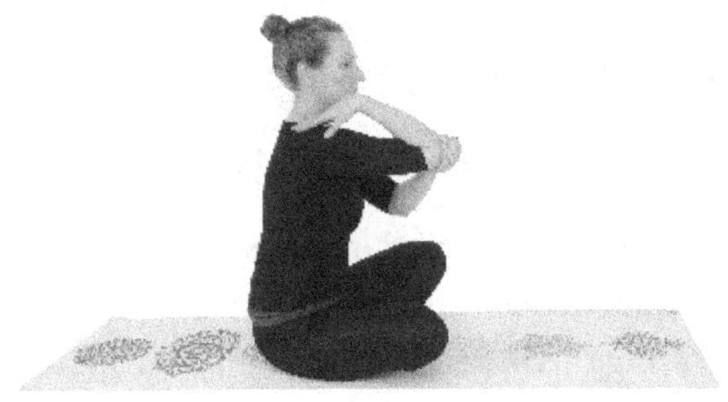

Practice: Touch with the left fingers the left shoulder, and with the right hand support the upper left arm. The left arm should be parallel to the ground on starting position. Rotate the bent left elbow in a full circle so that both lower arm and hand rotate together. The left fingers should be barely loose on the left shoulder so they move past while rotating. Slowly lower the left arm and repeat the same with the right side. Practice slowly 5-8 times clockwise and anticlockwise.

Breathing: Inhale on upward movement. Exhale on downward movement.

Awareness: On breathing, the rotation of the elbow joint and on maintaining the upper arm steady.

14. Shoulder Movement Up and Down – Skakthi Vikasaka

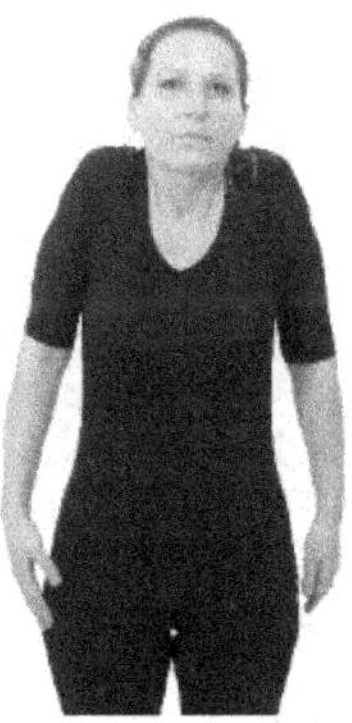

Practice: Elevate shoulders up toward the ears trying to touch the ears. This is the upward movement and is called elevation. When bringing the shoulders down, try to press them further down from the normal position. This is the downward movement and is called depression.

Breathing: Inhale on elevation. Exhale on depression.

Awareness: On breathing and the shoulders' movement.

Note: This practice can be performed in either standing or any cross-legged seated position. If practicing while seating, then position hands on the knees and by extending them, gently push shoulders up. In either position, move the shoulders without any strain or tension in the abdomen area.

Neck Movements

In pregnancy, naturally many women attract thyroid disorders and neck movements are considered beneficial for that, as well as the stretching of the neck muscles to relieve from stiffness arising from bad posture while feeding the baby in the postnatal period.

For those suffering from vertigo, it is advisable to practice with eyes open. If dizziness still occurs, practitioner should take a few moments to breath with eyes open until full sensations are back in the head and neck. In such case, practitioner should stop performing the neck movements at least for that day.

TIP: For those who may feel dizziness during these practices, they could rub their palms to generate heat for a few seconds and transfer that positive heat to their closed eyes by cupping them. When feeling comfortable they can slowly open eyes.

15. Neck Movements – Greeva Sanchalana

Practice: Sit up straight in a comfortable cross-legged position, with shoulders relaxed and hands resting in the knees. Eyes should remain open during the practice, however would-be-mums suffering from nausea or dizziness can keep them closed, and after finishing the neck movements can take 1-2 breaths with eyes closed, rub the palms vigorously and cuff the eyes for a few moments before opening the eyes to continue with practice. This is the starting position.

Variation 1: Left to Right

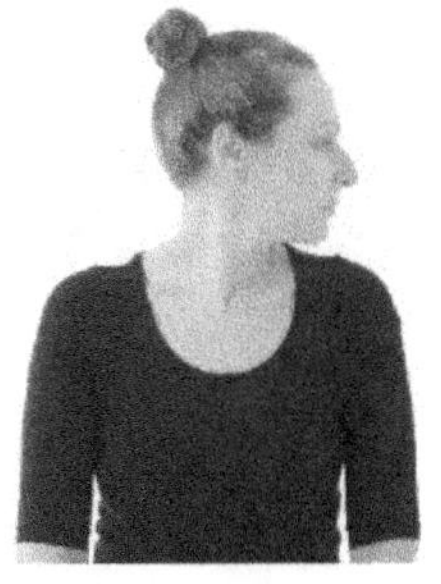

From starting position, inhale at the center, exhale while turning to the right shoulder. Inhale to return to the center, exhale while turning to the left shoulder. This is 1 round. Can practice 3-5 rounds. Practice can be slow or medium speed, as we need to avoid jerky body movements. Every time feel the stretch in the neck muscles and the loosening of the neck joints.

Breathing: Inhale while coming to the center. Exhale while turning to the left or right side.

Variation 2: Up and Down

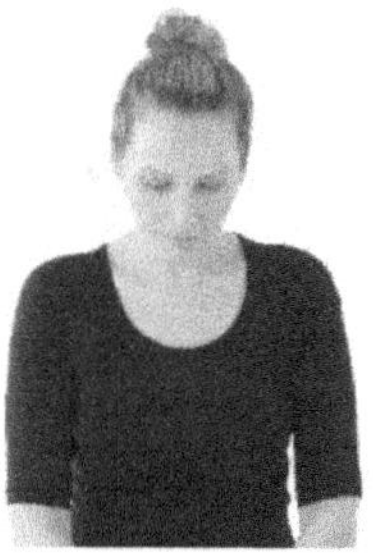

From starting position, inhale with neck in upright position, and on exhalation drop chin to the chest. Inhale and move head up and backwards without any strain and exhale to move head forward trying to touch the chest with the chin. Repeat 10 times, and on every move feel the stretch in the front and back neck muscles and the loosening of the vertebrae.

Breathing: Inhale on moving head up and backwards. Exhale on bring head down and forward.

Variation 3: Side to Side

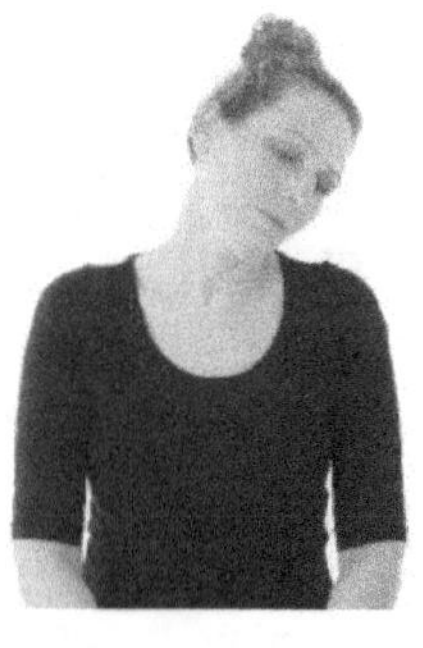

Practice: Sit up straight in a comfortable cross-legged position, with shoulders relaxed, hands resting in the knees and eyes closed. Inhale with neck in upright position and face looking forward and on exhalation slowly tilt head to the right trying to touch the shoulder with the ear; left shoulder should attempt to slightly move downwards for maximum stretch. Inhale as you return to the center and from center exhale to move the head to the left side. This is 1 round. Can practice 3-5 rounds, and on every move feel the stretch in the side neck muscles and the loosening of the joints.

Breathing: Inhale on the upward movement. Exhale on the downward movement.

Variation 4: Full Rotation

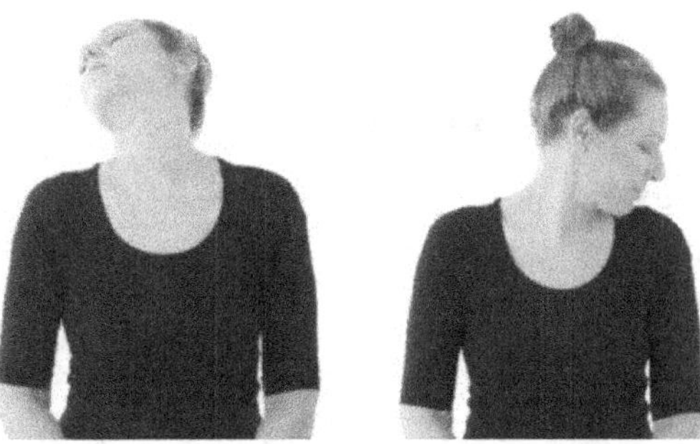

From starting position, inhale with neck dropped forward while trying to touch the chin to the chest. On exhalation, slowly rotate the head backwards passing by the shoulder, to the back of the neck and to the other side until a full circle is complete. Inhale at the center to repeat rotation. This is 1 round. Can practice 3-5 rounds clockwise and anti-clockwise. On every rotation feel the stretch in the neck muscles and the loosening of the neck joints. No pressure or extra stretch should be forced to the rotation. Move should be natural according to vertebrae capacity and head gravity; rotation should be slow, circular, gentle and comfortable.

Modification: Those suffering from neck injuries or neck pain, or those who experience nausea and dizziness, should only practice Half Rotation. From starting position, practice a semi-circle while exhaling to the right.

With continuous movement, inhale on half rotating the neck to the left, exhale to complete half rotation to the right. Repeat 3-5 times on each side and on every rotation feel the stretch in the neck muscles and the loosening of the neck joints.

Breathing: Inhale on rotating head backward and to the side. Exhale on rotating head downward.

Awareness: On breathing and neck movement or rotation.

Contraindications: Those suffering from high blood pressure should avoid doing this practice. Those who suffer from vertigo should try the half rotation with eyes open, and after completing practice should return to starting position with eyes remaining open and neck straight until they have full sensations in the head and neck.

16. Standing Pelvic Rotation

In addition to Pawanmuktasana Part 1, pelvic rotations are not only a great warm-up exercise but also a cooling down between practices and at the end of the practice.

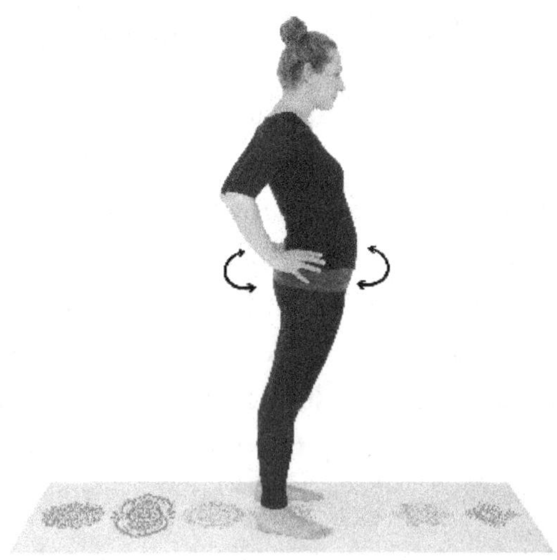

Practice: From a standing position with the feet slightly apart and the spine erect, place the palms of the hands on top of the hips or on the waist area and start rotating the pelvis area in slow and controlled 360° degree circle. A full circle is 1 round. Can practice 5-8 rounds clockwise and anti-clockwise.

Modification: For those with severe back pain or imbalance on this position, can practice half rotation to the back for 5-8 rounds and equal rounds to the front.

Breathing: Inhale on rotating pelvis backward and to the side. Exhale on rotating pelvis forward and to the center.

Awareness: Physical – on breathing and pelvic rotation. Spiritual – on sacral (swadhisthana) chakra.

Pawanmuktasana Part 2

Those with major issues in the lumbar region have to be cautious when practicing. A modification for cautious practicing is to minimize the length of the motion of the legs. Any practitioner who is suffering from high blood pressure, serious heart conditions or back conditions such as, sciatica, slipped disc, lumbago, or hernia, peptic ulcer or had had abdominal surgery in that case Caesarean Section should not perform any of these practices, especially not without consulting a healthcare advisor.

With the following list of asanas tightness and tiredness in the lumbar area is relieved, while these practices are focusing on the digestive system and abdominal area. Very important during this pre-conception phase and the first year of motherhood is the core area as the fat deposits usually get stored around the waist and abdomen as well as the hip area. These fat deposits get burned and a practitioner can reduce weight in combination of a balanced nutrition. The abdomen organs maintain healthy and active, and is also excellent for reproductive system disorders. The digestive system strengthens up, and whether someone experiences indigestion, acidity, constipation, irregular bowl movement, excess gas, lack of appetite or diabetes can be also very beneficial. This group of asanas benefits the hip joints, knee joints, tones up the abdominal, lower back and spinal muscles. Can relieve tightness and tiredness and can restore freshness, especially if practiced early in the morning. These are excellent practices for correcting the fire element inside the body. These practices work on the core area which is related to stimulate and activate the solar plexus (manipura chakra) and can help those who are not so confident or courageous, and those who often feel anxious.

All of the following poses are on supine position. Can start with shavasana to physically relax the whole body and then bring awareness to breath and harmonize self before start practicing.

17. Raised Leg Pose – Padotthanasana

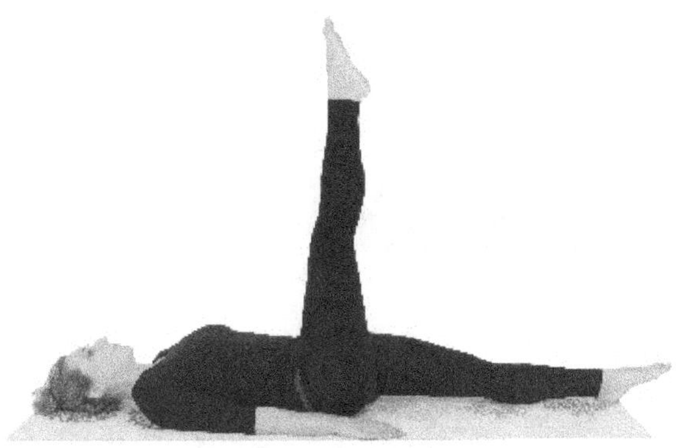

Practice: From Shavasana, bring legs closer together and the palms flat on the floor. This is the starting position. With inhalation, raise slowly left leg up to 90° degrees, with toes flexed and leg comfortably straight. The right leg should remain straight and grounded. Hold the position for 3-5 seconds (retain breathing) and with exhalation slowly bring left leg down. Practice 10 rounds per leg.

Modification: Those with weak back, instead of having grounded the extended leg, can bend the leg so the sole is flat on the ground and the knee is facing the ceiling.

Variation 1: Both legs together

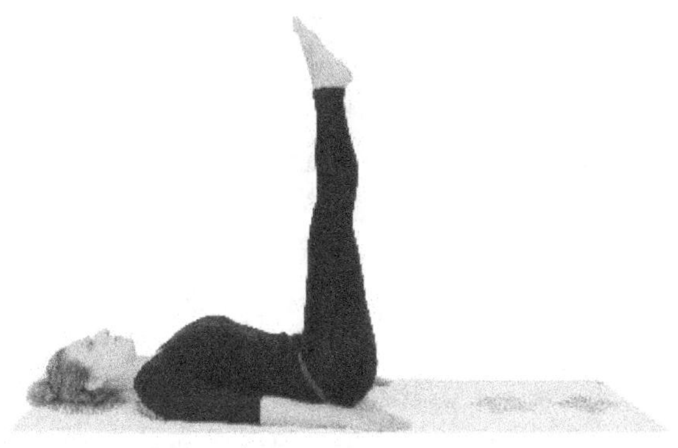

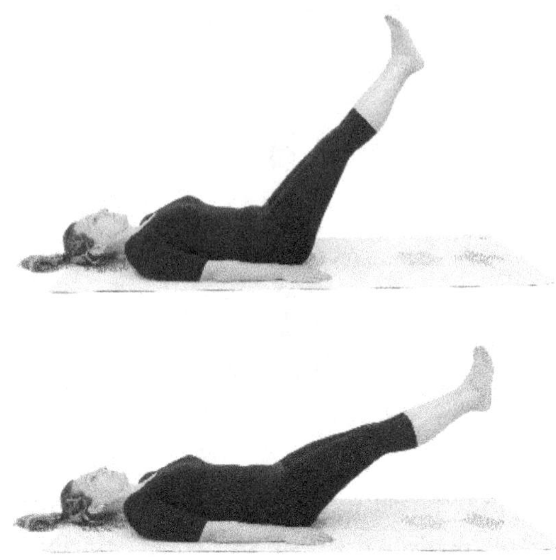

With inhalation, raise slowly both legs up to 90° or 45° or 30° degrees, with toes flexed and leg comfortably straight. Hold the position for 3-5 seconds (retain breathing) and with exhalation slowly bring left leg down. Practice 2 sets of 10 counts.

Variation 2: With the baby

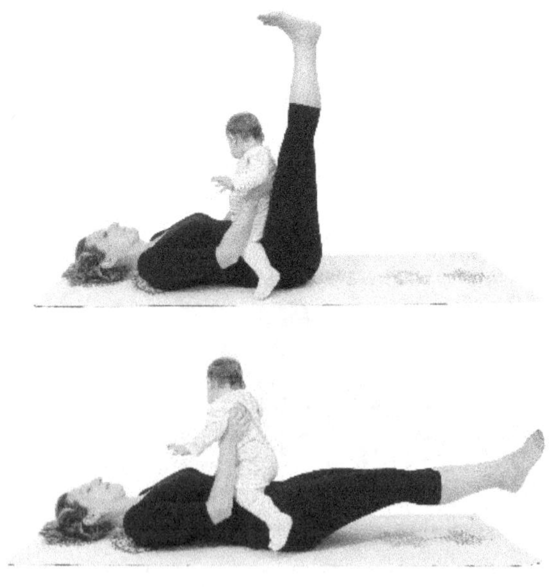

Similar to Variation 1. The hands should be holding the baby. The baby's weigh is making the practice more dynamic for the core and chest area.

Variation 3:

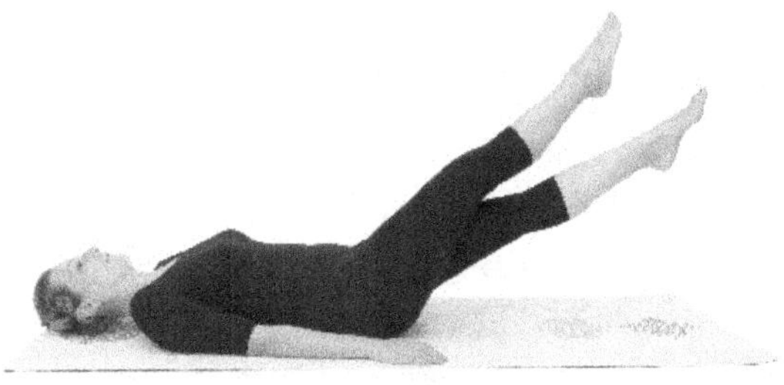

With continuous breathing perform the scissors where on a fast but steady move the legs open and close crosswise. Can move legs up and down when practicing or can keep them stable at 90° or 60° or 45° or 30° degrees. Advanced practitioners can go all the way down to 10° degrees. Can practice 2 sets of 10 counts up and down.

Breathing: Inhale on raising leg(s). Hold posture and breath. Exhale on lowering leg(s).

Awareness: On leg(s) stretching and breath-movement synchronization. Stage 2 and Stage 3 awareness should also be drawn to the muscular effort in the back and abdomen.

Note: To be practiced only from fourth trimester onwards and only if the body has completely recovered from childbirth.

18. Leg Rotation – Padachakrasana

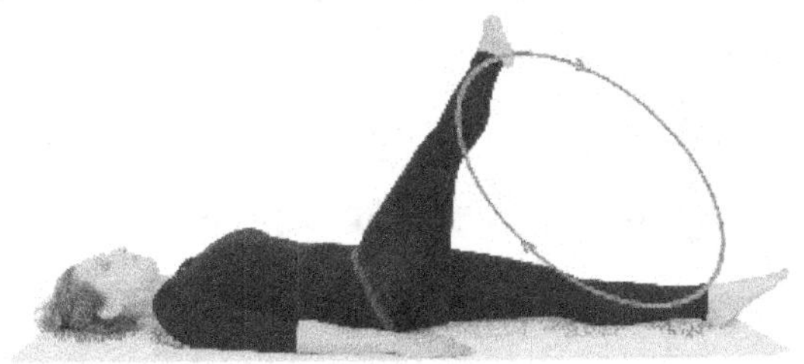

Variation 1: Single Leg Rotation

With inhalation, raise left leg to approximately 60° degrees, keeping the knee straight. Rotate the entire left leg in a large comfortable circle, where move should be done from the hip. The right leg should remain straight and in contact with the ground. The rotation should be continuous. Repeat the same with right leg. Practice for 10 rotations clockwise and 10 anticlockwise per leg.

Variation 2: Both Leg Rotation

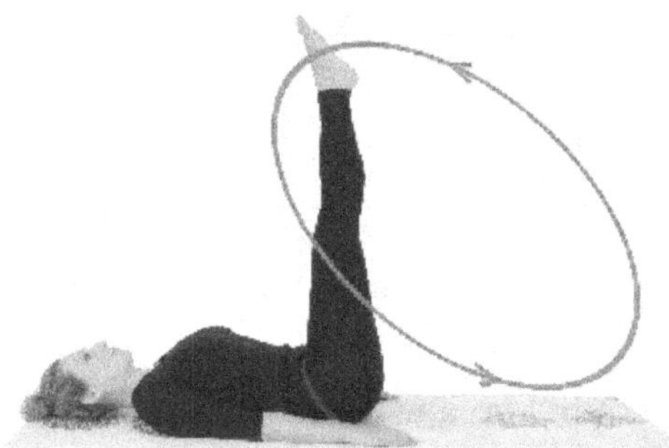

When rotating both legs, may have a strong effect and pressure on the lumbar region; can either position palms of the hands underneath the buttocks or further away from the body or place a soft blanket or towel under the lumbar. With inhalation, raise both legs keeping them together with knees straight. Rotate both legs in a comfortable circle, where move should be done from the hips. The rotation should be continuous without any strain. Practice for 5 rotations clockwise and 5 anticlockwise.

Breathing: Inhale on raising leg(s). Exhale on lowering leg(s).

Awareness: On leg(s) rotation and breath-movement synchronization from the hips with engaged core.

Precautions: Those suffering from high blood pressure or serious back conditions or sciatica should not practice this asana.

19. Cycling – Pada Sanchalanasana

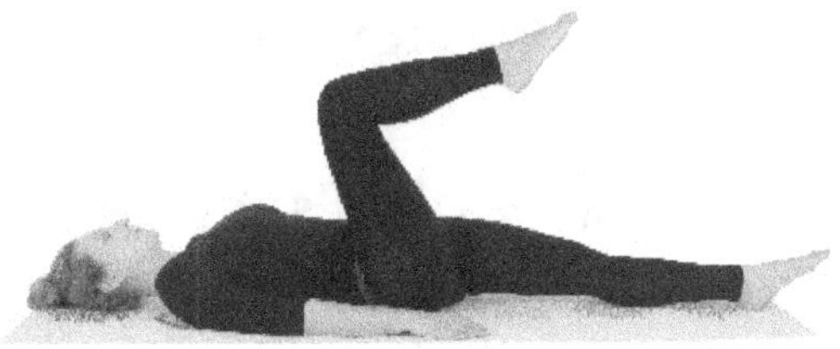

Variation 1: Single Leg Cycling

With inhalation, raise left leg with the knee bent and thigh closer to the chest. Straighten the leg on the forward movement, and bend it from the knee as it comes back toward the chest complete the cycling movement. The right leg should remain straight and in contact with the ground. The cycling to be continuous. Practice for 10 counts in forward direction and 10 counts in reverse direction per leg.

Variation 2: Alternate Legs Cycling – Normal Breathing

Raise both legs together with knees bent and thighs closer to the chest. Practice alternate leg cycling by extending the knees on the forward movement and bending them on the backward movement.

Practice for 10 counts in forward direction and 10 in backward direction.

Variation 3: Both Legs Cycling

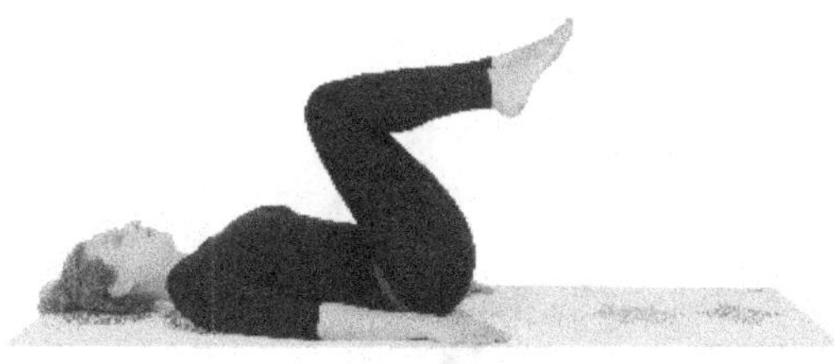

With inhalation, raise both legs together with knees bent and thighs closer to the chest. As the legs lower forward shall be straight until the legs are as close to the ground as comfortable – but not touching the ground; and as legs come back towards the chest, knees shall be bent to complete the cycling movement. The cycling to be continuous. Practice for 10 counts in forward direction and 10 counts in reverse per leg.

Breathing: Inhale on straightening leg(s). Exhale on bending leg(s) to the chest.

Awareness: Synchronization of breath and movement, particularly on reverse cycling while practicing. At relaxation after asana performance, focus on the breath and the abdomen, hip, thighs and lower back sensation.

20. Leg Lock Pose – Supta Pawanmuktasana

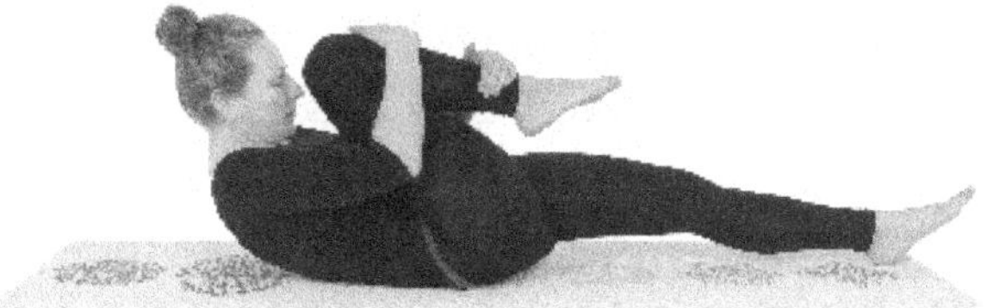

Variation 1: One Leg Lock

Bend left knee, interlock fingers, clasp hands on the shin and bring knee closer to the chest. Inhale and on exhalation lift head and shoulders trying to touch the knee with the nose. Hold the position and breathing for a few seconds and slowly come back to the floor with the knees bent. The right leg should be straight and on the ground. Repeat the same with right leg. Practice 3-5 times with each leg.

Variation 2: Both Legs Lock

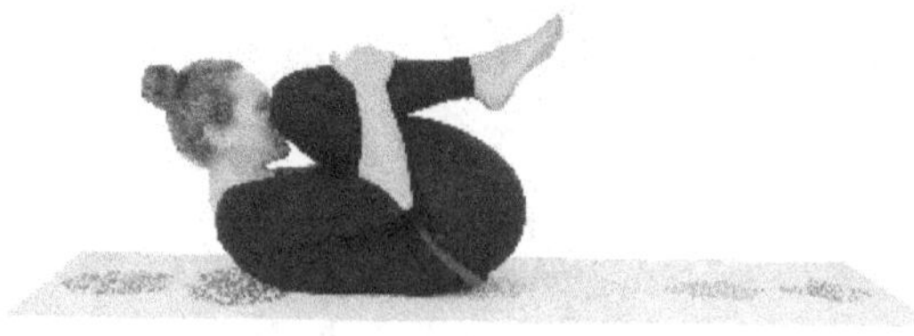

Bend both knees, interlock fingers, clasp hands on the shins with normal breathing. Exhale to bring the knees closer to the chest, raise the head and shoulders and gently without any neck strain bring the nose as close and between the knees. Hold the position and breathing for a few seconds and slowly come back to the floor with the knees bent. Practice 3-5 times.

Variation 3: With the baby

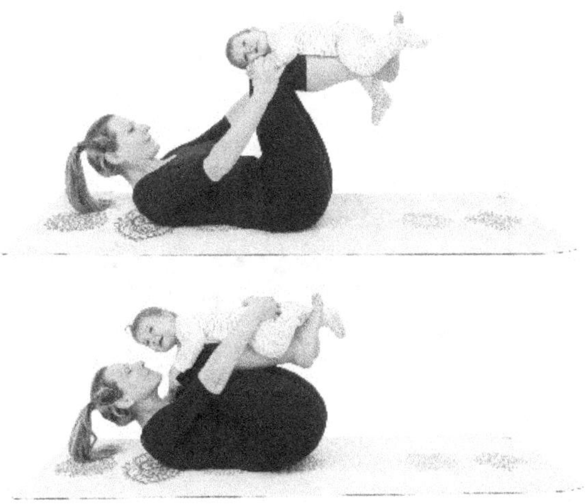

During the first year of motherhood, this asana can be practiced with the baby on top of the shins to strengthen the abdomen area. Carefully position the baby on top of the shins with legs raised at table top position, and with caution bring legs forward to the chest on inhalation. On exhalation extend legs away from the body returning to original position, where knees should be on the same line with hips. Practice becomes more advanced and challenging as the baby grows and weight is increased. Practice for 3-5 counts or as many it feels comfortable.

Breathing: Inhale on bending legs to the chest. Exhale on extending legs to table top position.

Awareness: On breath-movement synchronization and the abdominal pressure; not dropping the baby.

Precautions: Must be aware of any strain in the lower back and should not be practiced if suffering from back conditions, such as lumbago, sciatica and slipped disk. Not to be practiced if suffering from high blood pressure.

Note: Pushing one knee to the chest will stretch the thigh area. The knees to the chest will stretch the thigh and lumbar area. When practicing with the baby, should always be cautious on baby movements as well, to avoid any injuries for both mother and baby.

21. Sleeping Abdominal Stretch – Supta Udarakarshanasana

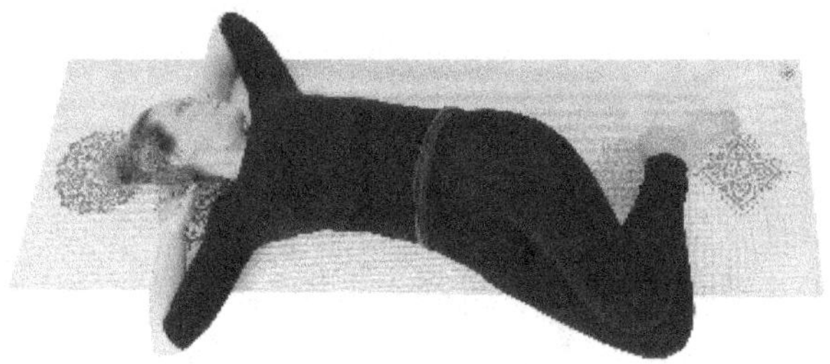

Practice:

From Shavasana, interlock fingers of both hands below the head with the elbows touching the floor. Keep the knees together and bent in front of the body with the heels in front and closer to the buttocks. Inhale and on exhalation slowly bring both knees down towards to the ground of the left side and at the same time turn head to the right side. Breathe normally for 2-3 breaths. Inhale back to the center. Exhale to the right side to repeat the same with head looking to the left side. Practice for 5 times on each side.

Variations:

- If tension needs to be released around the sacrum, keep feet approximately 60 cm from the buttocks.

- If tension needs to be released around the thoracic, keep feet closer to the buttocks.

- If focus of the practice is to activate the cardiac plexus, keep feet touching the buttocks or as close as possible.

Breathing: Inhale in starting position. Exhale on pushing knees to the ground. Hold breathing when knees are on the ground. Inhale while bringing bent legs back to the center.

Awareness: On breath and on relaxation of the back, arms and shoulders.

Benefits: Aim of this twist is for maximum stretch on the paraspinal and abdominal muscles.

Note: When moving by 3 cm each time the feet closer to the buttocks, each vertebra gets worked out, making the whole spinal column more flexible.

22. Universal Spinal Twist – Shava Udarakarshanasana

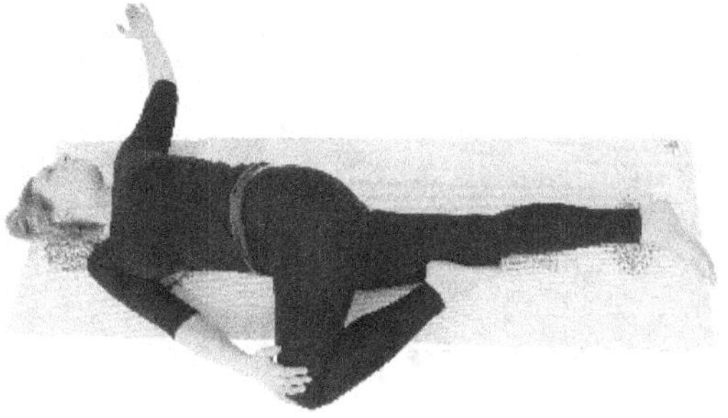

Practice:

From Shavasana, inhale and stretch both arms out to the sides of shoulders. On exhalation bend left knee with the sole of the foot on the ground and with the right hand press the knee down toward the right side of the body. The left arm should be stretched out to the side at shoulder level. Shoulder should be as close as possible to the ground – if can't touch the ground, and the head should be turned to the left with the gaze fixed at the middle finger of the extended left hand. Aim of this twist is for maximum stretch on the side of the body and intercostal muscles. Hold the position for as long as it feels comfortable by slow and deep breathing. To return to original position, bring head and knee to the center, stretch right arm open to the side and straighten the left leg. Repeat the same with right leg and opposite hand. Practice for 3 counts with each leg. On every count, try to hold the position by a few extra seconds.

Variation:

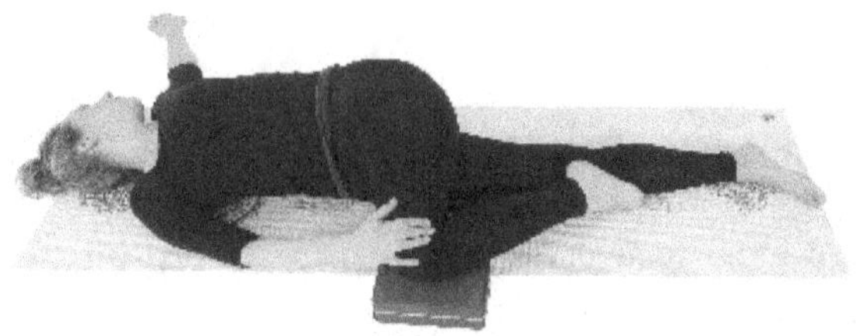

Practitioner can make use of a support system under the bent knee – such as a yoga block, a cushion or folded blanket if needed. Can also use a folded blanket or soft cushion under the shoulder of the extended arm to help grounding.

Breathing: Inhale in starting position. Exhale on pushing the knee to the ground. Slow and deep breathing during the twist. Inhale while bringing body back to the center. Exhale on strengthening the leg.

Awareness: On breath and on relaxation of the back, arms and shoulders.

Precautions: If practice becomes painful, should be stopped, as it can realign the hip joint.

23. Boat Pose – Naukasana

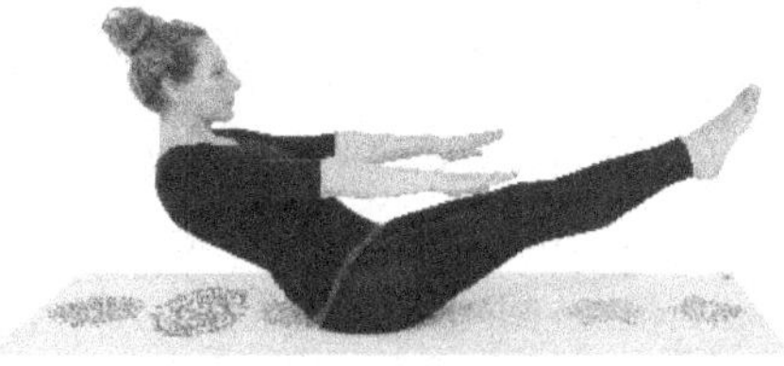

Practice: This is a practice only for Postnatal period and after complete recovery. From Shavasana, hands can either rest on the floor or on top of the thighs. Inhale deeply, hold breathing and raise legs, arms, shoulders, head and trunk off the ground. The arms to be in one line with the toes, palms facing down, gaze fixed on the toes. Hold position for 3 to 5 or more comfortable counts while tensing the abdominal muscles. Lower body spontaneously (but carefully not to hit the back of the head) to return to starting position before exhaling. Relax in Shavasana for a few abdominal breaths before resuming practice for next round. Practice for 5 rounds.

Modification: Clench the fists, squeeze the whole body and hold the raised position for 20-30 seconds for beginners, and longer for advanced practitioners.

Variation: With the Baby

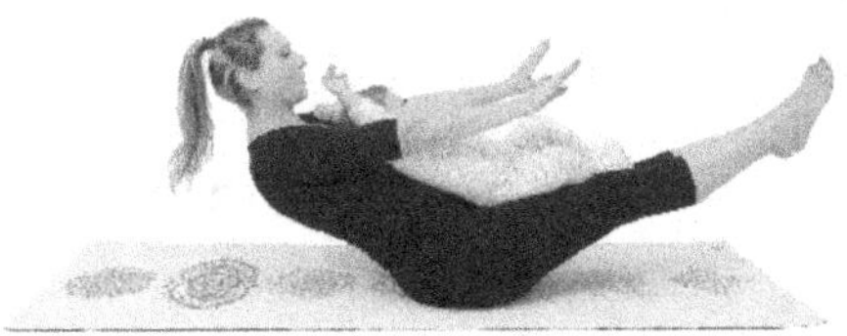

Can be practiced at fourth trimester and during the first year of motherhood with the baby on top, either facing mummy's face or the ceiling. Caution must be on the correct positioning of the body and the baby not to fall and get injured.

Breathing: Inhale before raising the body. Hold breathing while raising, tensing and lowering the body.

Exhale in the supine position.

Awareness: On breath, movement and tensing of the body; not dropping the baby.

Benefits: Stimulates the muscular, digestive, circulatory, nervous and endocrine systems

Note: Body needs to drop spontaneously because with this practice the store house of the prana energy gets activated which is located in the abdomen area, called the Pranic Center. When these energies get activated and body automatically drops down, these energies get distributed to the body evenly and nicely and bring to the physical body a relaxing effect. Brings suddenly a great amount of energy in the body and activates the whole nervous system. Beware of not hitting the head while dropping spontaneously to the floor.

Pawanmuktasana Part 3

The following list of asanas is particularly focusing to the pelvic floor area, organs and muscles. Any disorders to menstrual cycle, infertility, reproductive hormones and in general the endocrine function can be improved and lungs and heart can be activated.

Would-be-mums should avoid practicing, but if they choose to practice they should use cushions for support.

24. Pulling the Rope – Rajju Karshanasana

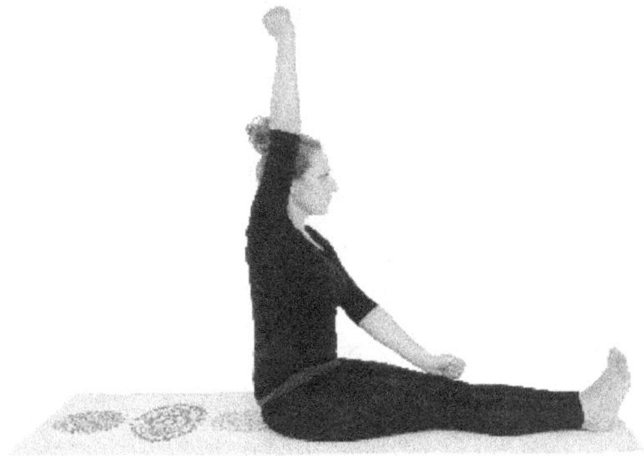

Practice: Sit in Base Position and place the hands on the knees, visualize a well where you are about to pull the rope. Inhale to lift up right arm pulling the rope as high as possible, with the elbow straight and eyes looking upward. Exhale to slowly bring the right arm down, applying pressure like you are lowering a heavy object where you should feel pressure on biceps, and eyes to follow the downward movement. Practice alternate arms for 10 counts each.

Breathing: Inhale to raise the arm. Exhale to lower the arm.

Awareness: On breath, movement and upper back/ shoulder muscles stretch.

Benefits: Loosens the shoulder joints, stretches upper back and shoulder muscles, firm the breast. When arm comes down you will feel a stretching effect in the side of the breasts connecting to the armpit and the tissues around the breasts will function properly. Therefore, this practice is related to the breast health as well as the toning of the hands region whereas all nerves around these areas get stimulated.

Note: This practice can be done during pregnancy with spine rested on a wall and legs apart on second trimester, and wider on the third trimester.

25. Dynamic Spinal Twist – Gatyatmak Meru Vakrasana

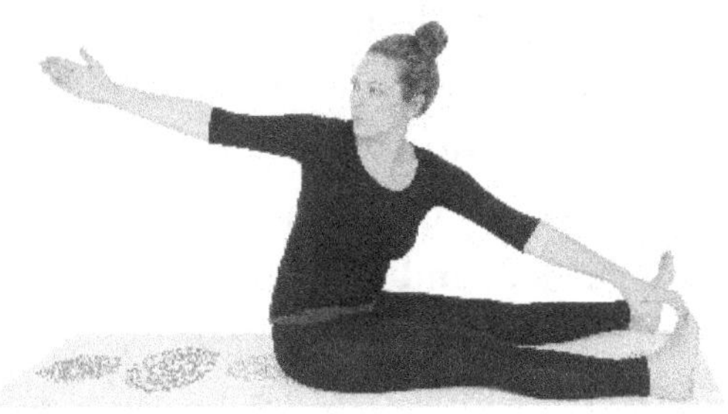

Practice: Sit with both legs outstretched as far apart as comfortable. With the arms stretched sideways at the shoulder level, twist to the right and with left hand touch the right big toe. Turn the head right and gaze at the right extended hand. Try to keep both arms straight and aligned. Twist to the other side by changing the hands; right hand to touch the left big toe, head turned to the left gazing the left outstretched hand. This is 1 round. Practice for 10 rounds.

Breathing: Inhale to the center. Exhale to on twisting for greater spine flexion.

Awareness: On breath synchronization with the movement.

Benefits: Relaxes from back stiffness, increases spine flexion.

Precautions: Should be avoid if suffering from back conditions.

Note: Round after round can increase the speed of movement making sure there is no rounding on the back or bending from the back. The whole movement should be from the hip joint only.

26. Churning the Mill – Chakki Chalanasana

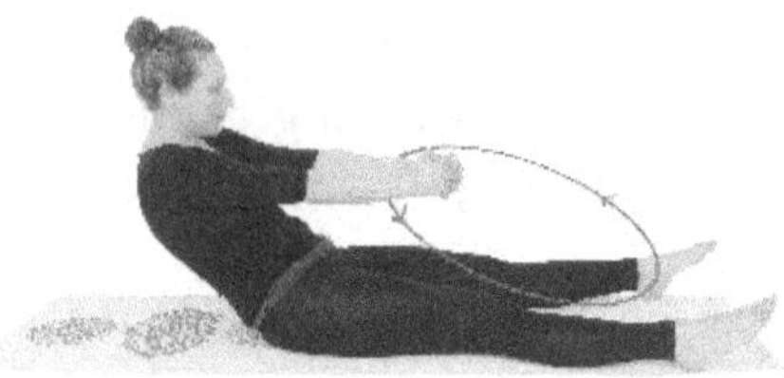

Practice: Sit with both legs outstretched as far apart as comfortable. Interlock the fingers with arms stretched in front of the chest; spine must be erect. From the hip joint slightly lean forward with the interlocked fingers to the center of the legs distance. At this position should feel the stretch on the inner thighs. Start making the rotation to the left where the hands pass above the left toes and swing backwards. On the forward movement pass the hands above the right toes and come back to the center. Practice 5-10 rounds clockwise and 5-10 anticlockwise.

Breathing: Inhale on backward movement. Exhale on forward movement.

Awareness: On breath synchronization with the movement.

Benefits: Great practice to tone up nerves, muscles and organs of the pelvis and abdomen area. Menstrual cycle regulator.

27. Rowing the Boat – Nauka Sanchalanasana

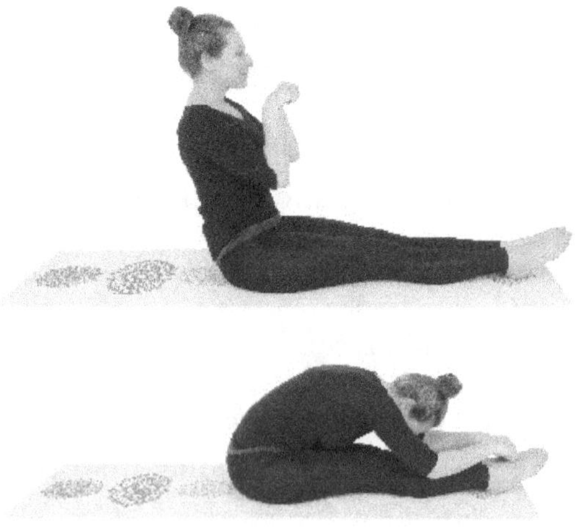

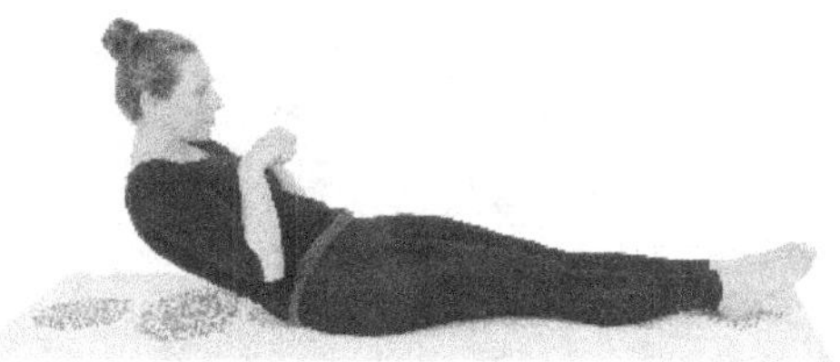

Practice: Sit with spine erect, both legs straight in front of the body and make a fist with the hands where palms are facing down. Exhale and bend forward from the hip joint and straighten the arms. Inhale and lean back from the hip joint and bend the hands back towards the chest. During the forward and backward movements, the hands should make a full circle. Practice for 10 rounds clockwise and 10 anticlockwise.

Breathing: Inhale to lean back. Exhale to bend forward.

Awareness: On breath, movement and focus on lower back, hips, and pelvic area.

Benefits: Loosens the shoulder joints, stretches upper back and shoulder muscles, firm the breast. When arm comes down you will feel a stretching effect in the side of the breasts connecting to the armpit and the tissues around the breasts will function properly. Therefore, this practice is related to the breast health as well as the toning of the hands region whereas all nerves around these areas get stimulated.

28. Chopping Wood – Kashtha Takshanasana

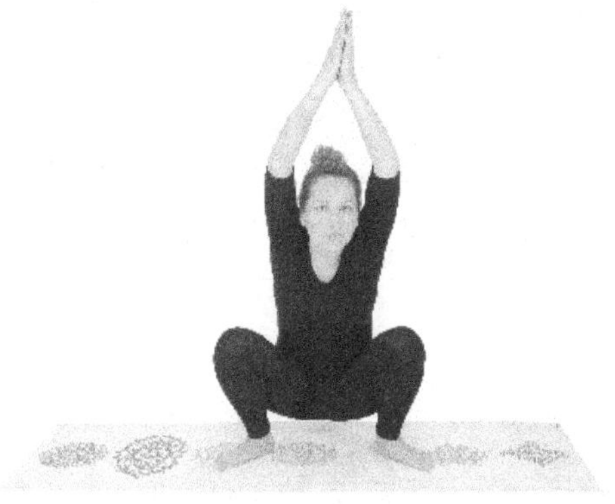

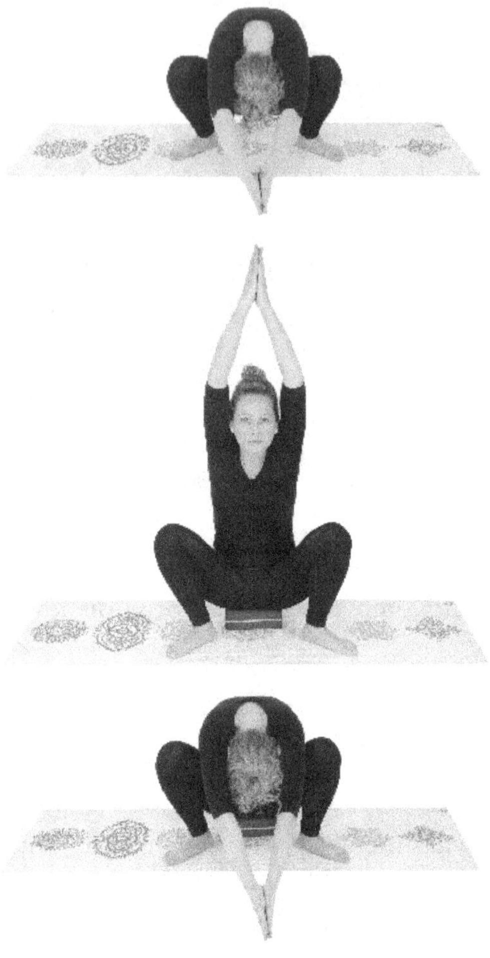

Practice: Squat with the feet flat on the floor approximately 45 cm apart. Elbows should be positioned on the inner knees. If feeling pressure on the knees, you may need to raise buttocks higher, in such case use a double cushion to sit on or a yoga block. Interlock fingers with straightened arms, keep them down and near the floor, look down the fingers. On inhalation raise straightened arms above and behind the head with spine erect. Look up the interlocked fingers. On exhalation, bring straightened arms rapidly down near the floor in between the feet by making the sound "Ha!" Visualize you are actually chopping the wood. Practice for 10 counts.

Modification: Can sit on a yoga blog or cushions.

Breathing: Inhale on upward movement. Exhale on downward movement.

Awareness: On breath synchronization with the movement and stretching of the shoulders and upper back muscles.

Benefits: Physical – Breast tissues and nerves get activated for maximum breast health. During menstrual cycle progesterone hormone can cause breast stiffness and soreness and this practice can help overcome symptoms. Loosens up the pelvic girdle and tones up the pelvic muscles. Activates the inaccessible muscles of the shoulder blades, works the shoulder joints and upper back muscles. Spiritual – Helps to release aggravation and lighten the mood.

Precautions: Not to be practiced by people with knee problems or sciatica.

Note: Can be performed during pregnancy only if practitioner was practicing this asana daily and before conception. Otherwise there will be excess pressure and reversal force applied on the belly. General note is not to perform this during pregnancy.

29. Salutation Pose – Namaskarsana

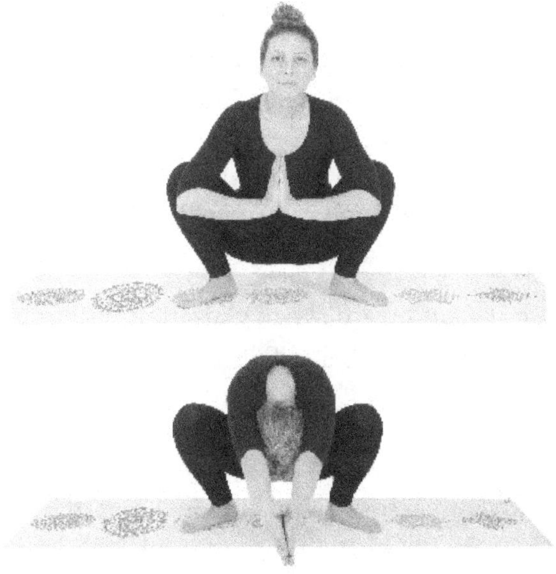

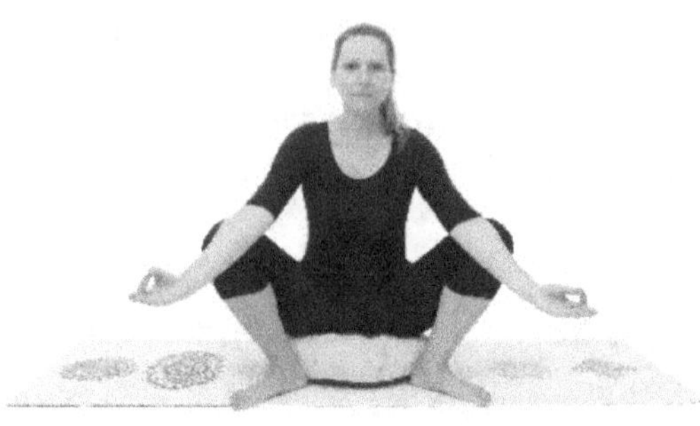

Practice: Squat with the feet flat on the floor approximately 60 cm apart. Elbows should be positioned on the inner knee. Bring the palms together into Namaste Mudra keeping the hands down, and look down. On inhalation raise head up, bring the hands into the prayer in front of the chest, the elbows to push the knees away from each other and look up. On exhalation bring head downwards while extending the hands down by maintaining the anjali mudra throughout the whole practice. Practice for 10 counts.

Modification (Second and Third Trimester): Take the support of a cushion to sit on. Make sure the thighs are away from the belly to avoid any hitting during practice. If feeling pressure on the knees, practitioner may need to raise buttocks even higher with an additional cushion. Inhale to bring hands on anjali mudra as close it feels comfortable in front of the chest area. During exhalation, the hands should be lowered to the level belly is not receiving any pressure.

Breathing: Inhale on hands upward movement. Exhale on hands downward movement.

Awareness: Physical – on breath synchronization with the movement and cautious to avoid hitting the belly. Spiritual – on sacral (swadhisthana) chakra and root (mooladhara).

Benefits: Opens the pelvic region and prepares the body for childbirth. Can be helpful for indigestion, constipation and flatulence. Stretches, strengthens and loosens the hips, knees and ankles. Can prevent cramps as it stretches the calves and the thighs. Relaxes the upper back, shoulder and neck muscles. Helps baby to come to correct position for birth.

Precautions: Should not be practiced by people with knee problems or on the first trimester. It can be challenging to practice for those who are not used to squatting or sitting on the floor. Avoid this asana if placenta previa1F[2], cervical stitch, hemorrhoids, breech baby2F[3], premature dilation of the cervix, preterm labor.

30. Wind Releasing Pose – Vayu Nishkasana

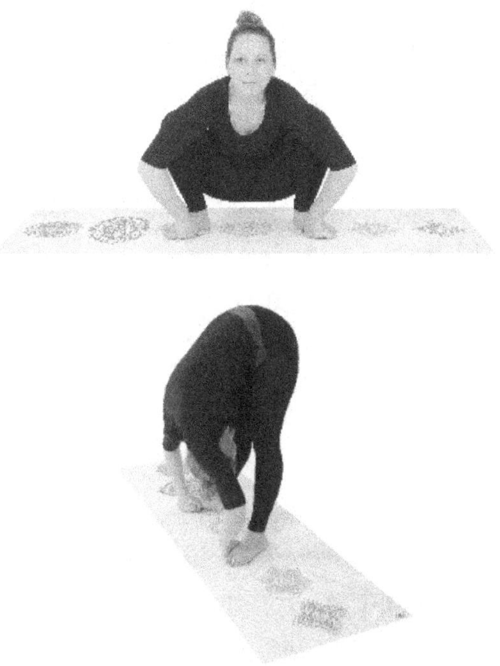

Practice: Start with the squatting position with the feet flat on the floor approximately 60 cm apart. Place the hands under the arch of the sole with the thumbs above. The upper arms should gently push out the knees with the elbows slightly bent. On inhalation slowly move the head back, fix gaze

---

[2] When placenta covers (partially or totally) the opening of the cervix. Can cause severe bleeding during pregnancy and delivery.

[3] If baby has not come to position with head down after 35 or 36 gestation week

upward and take 2 breaths there. On exhalation, slowly lift the buttocks up, try to straighten the knees and bring the head forward towards the knees. Hold the position for a few seconds with normal breathing and focus on flexing the spine and spinal bend. Do not strain, as it may overstretch muscles or ligaments of the back. On inhalation, return to the original position. Practice for 10 continuous rounds with normal breathing, at the end slowly release the hands.

Breathing: Inhale on squatting. Exhale on lifting up.

Awareness: On breath synchronization with the movement.

Benefits: Stretches and flexes the groin, compresses the back of the neck, relaxed the upper back and shoulder muscles. Tones up nerves and muscles on thighs, knees, shoulders, arms and neck. Massages pelvic organs and muscles. Stretches and tones up all spinal nerves when all the vertebrae and joints are pulled away from each other for balanced pressure between them. Stretches the whole spine, arms and leg muscles. Helps releasing accumulation of gas in the alimentary canal.

Precautions: Should not be practiced by people with high blood pressure, arteriosclerosis, knee problems or sciatica.

Note: Some people can only micro-bent the knees. On every round attempt more straightening of the knees and with regular practice will manage to completely straighten them. After practice sit on a comfortable meditative pose with closed eyes, hands on the knees, place awareness on navel or at the center of eyebrows and take a few breaths to relax. To relax the legs, practice Ankle Bending – Goolf Naman and Ankle Rotation – Goolf Chakra.

31. Crow Walking – Kauva Chalasana

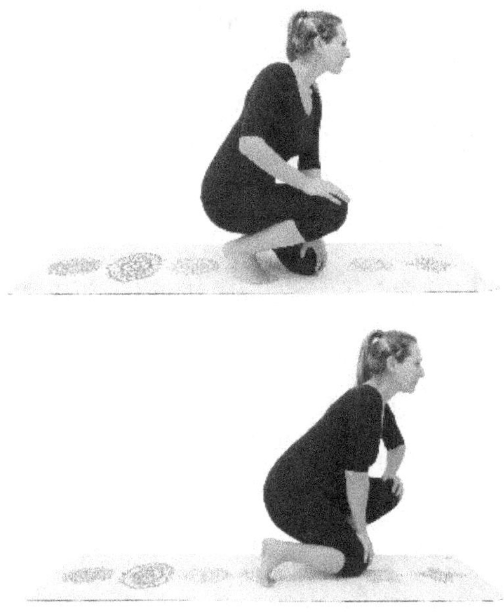

Practice: Start with the squatting position, feet should be as wide apart as it feels comfortable and stand on the toes, with buttocks above the heels. Place the palms on the knees. In that position, look forward and start walking in straight direction where left foot is coming out, right knee is coming inwards and towards the left foot. Walk either on the toes or the soles of the feet. If new practitioner, can walk with whichever feels easier for a gentle movement and after mastering the practice, walk with the most difficult. The squat whole movement should give the experience of pressure in the abdomen. Practice for 3 rounds minimum walking up and down on the mat, or as many as 50 steps. After practice relax in Shavasana.

Variation: While moving can gently stretch the upper body looking over the left shoulder when the right knee comes on the ground, and the right shoulder when the left knee comes on the ground.

Breathing: Normal breathing, or synchronization of breath with movement: inhale to come to position, exhale to bring the knee to the ground, inhale to bring knee up, exhale to bring the other knee to the ground.

Awareness: Smoothing the movement while walking. After practice, come to Shavasana to rest and focus on the heartbeat and breathing, as well as the effects on the lower back, hips, knees, ankles.

Benefits: Legs preparatory asana for meditation asanas. Strengthens the knees, improves legs' blood circulation. Also helps remove constipation and massages internal pelvic organs.

Precautions: Should not be practiced by people with knee, ankles or toes problems and injuries.

Note: This practice is a preparatory one for pre-conception and should not be practiced during pregnancy. During pregnancy Karandavasana should be practiced instead.

Relaxation Asanas

Relaxation asanas should be performed before, during and after practicing to relax the tired body. Correct practicing of those requires conscious relaxation of all body muscles, which is difficult to achieve considering the ease of these asanas in physical terms.

32. Corpse Pose – Shavasana

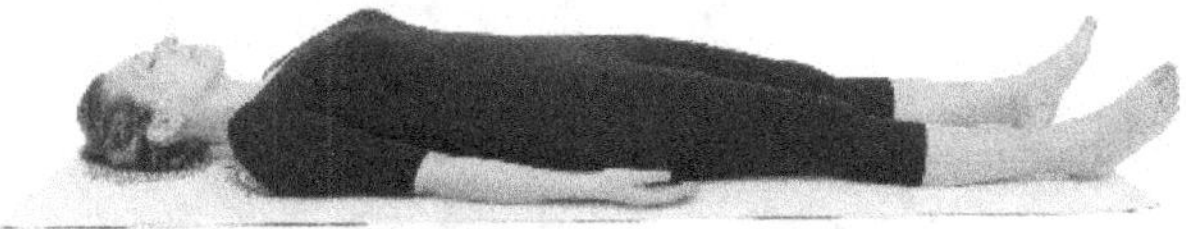

Practice: Lie on supine position with the arms slightly away from the body, at about 15 cm. The palms facing upwards with the fingers relaxed. Adjust feet to be slightly apart from each other, lie down comfortably and close the eyes. The head and spine should be aligned, and the head should be comfortably in a way that face looks up without falling to either sides. Relax the body on that position without any physical movement. Focus on natural breath and gradually feel it rhythmic and relaxed. When practice is consumed, become aware of the physical body and surroundings, and gently release the pose by moving smoothly the toes and fingers. When ready, with the eyes closed and the support of the right hand, sit up from the left side.

Modification 1:

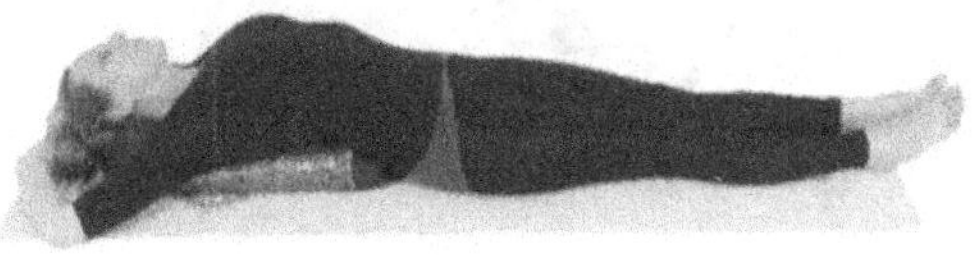

During the first and second trimester, should use a bolster along the spine to lift up the body. During the third trimester should have a bigger lift of about 20% inclination on the upper body, to avoid compressing the inferior vena cava. If it feels comfortable, position the hands behind or above the head. Otherwise, position the hands next to the body with the palms facing the ceiling.

Modification 2:

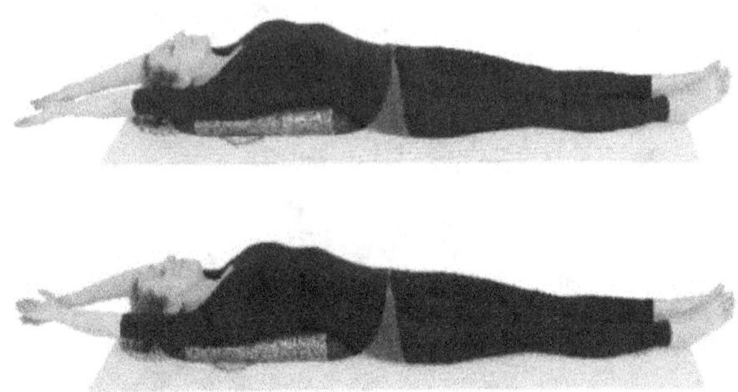

Similar to Modification 1, extend the arms above the head and while on bolster, stretch the upper body. Position the palms either facing up the ceiling, or one on top of the other, whichever feels more comfortable.

Modification 3:

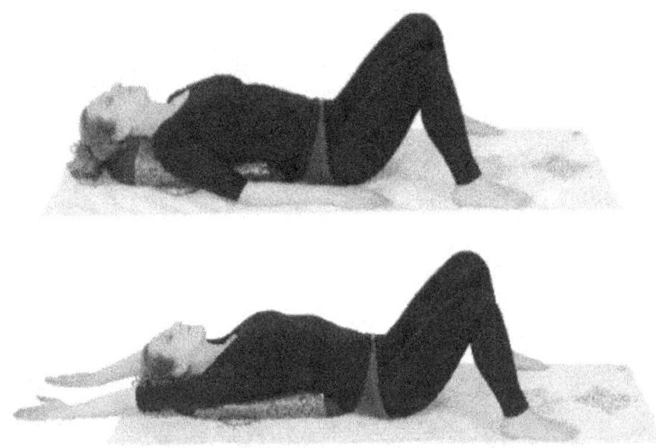

Similar to Modification 1 and 2, bend the knees wide apart to release tension from lumbar area.

Breathing: Normal breathing. Can also count backwards from number 27, where mentally repeating, "I am breathing in 27, I am breathing out 27, I am breathing in 26, I am breathing out 26, I am breathing in 25, I am breathing out 25…" and so on until zero. If the mind loses the counting, should start from the beginning, at 27. Aim of this practice is to connect the mind with the breath for a few minds in order to relax the physical body.

Duration: Between asanas, 1 or 2 minutes to relax the body. For relaxation and Yoga Nidra, depending to time availability.

Awareness: Physical; first to relax the body and then on breathing. Spiritual; third Eye (Ajna) chakra.

Benefits: Between practices should be practiced to relax the mind and body. Generally, it develops physical and mental awareness, relieves muscles tension, lowers blood pressure, reduces insomnia.

Precautions: During the pregnancy, especially from second trimester onwards, should not practice Shavasana or any other supine position, to avoid compression of Inferior Vena Cava. It can be practiced if modified to inclined positioning of minimum 20% of the upper back, neck and head with the support of pillows or hard bolster.

Note: Can use a thin pillow behind the head for more comfort if needed. The body should remain still throughout the whole practice; a single movement can distract the practice. Typically, is considered the final resting pose. We have to use a support system of a cushion or a bolster on the lower back for two reasons: a) the back should not be flat on the ground; b) the body should be higher than the floor at this position so there will be not much effort on coming and releasing the position, and also no compression on the inferior vena cava.

33. Flapping Fish Pose – Matsya Kridasana

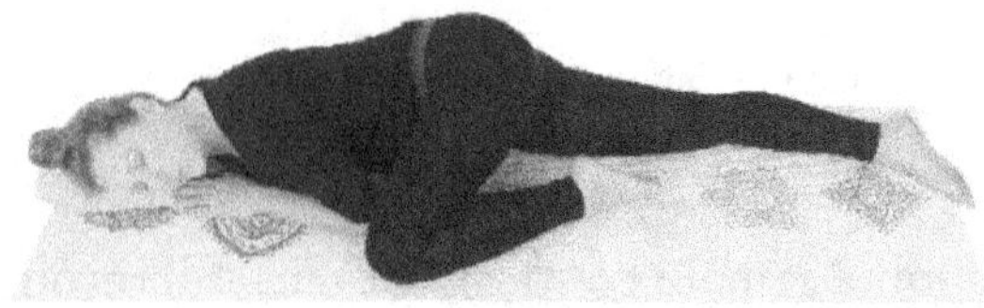

Practice: During the first trimester and usually around the end of fourth trimester if had a caesarian section, can lie on the stomach with the fingers interlocked under the head. Bend the left leg as close to the ribcage as possible. The right leg should remain straight and still. Rest the left elbow close to the left knee. Rest the right side of the head on or close to the crook of the right hand so head sits comfortably.

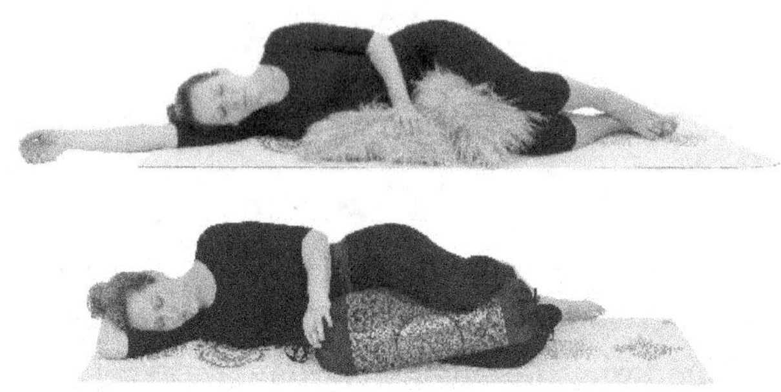

During the second and third trimester, lie on the left side with the fingers interlocked under the head, or extending the left arm and resting the head comfortably on the upper limb. Use the support of a cushion between the thighs and another cushion between the ground and the belly. Bend the knees or have them in a comfortable angle that does not compress the belly. Rest the right hand in front of the belly. Relax in one side for a few minutes and change sides.

Breathing: Normal breathing.

Duration: Between asanas, 1 or 2 minutes to relax the body from both sides. Equal amount of time should be given to both sides. For relaxation and Yoga Nidra, depending to time availability.

Awareness: Physical – first to relax the body and then on breathing. Spiritual – solar plexus (manipura) chakra.

Benefits: Stimulates the digestive system, can relieve from sciatic pain as it relaxes the nerves in the legs. It relaxes the perineum.

Note: The body should remain comfortable and still throughout the whole practice; a single movement can distract the practice. During the third trimester should avoid shavasana, instead, practice Matsya Kridasana for resting, relaxation, sleeping or practicing yoga nidra.

34. Reclined Butterfly Pose – Supta Baddhakonasana

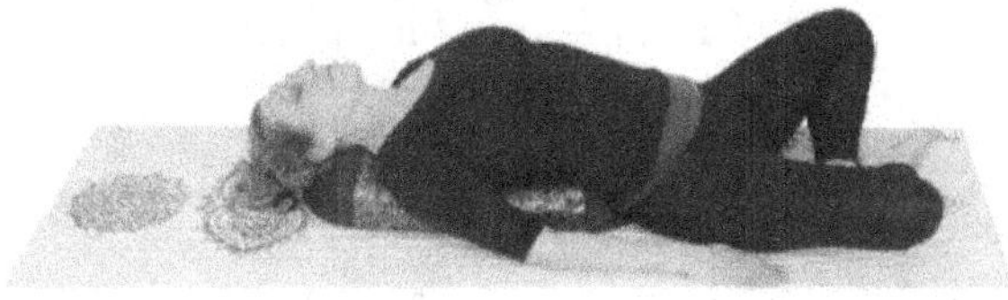

Practice: Sit on Sukhasana and place a cushion on the lower back to lie down on it. If it feels more comfortable, can use a long bolster along the spinal column. Adjust the position so the lumbar is on the cushion, the feet are comfortably positioned aiming for the knees to be closer to the ground. In any case, position must feel comfortable. Close the eyes and relax on that position.

Variation 1:

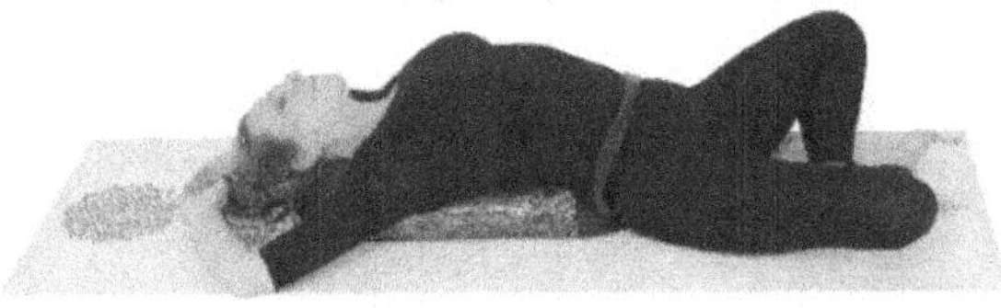

Can place the hands bent from the elbows behind the head with the palms facing the ceiling.

Variation 2:

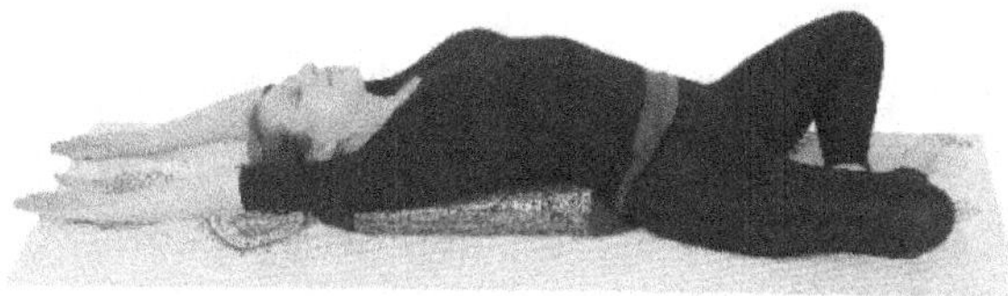

Can extend the arms backwards with the palms facing the ceiling for maximum stretch on arms, shoulder blades and rib cage.

Breathing: Normal breathing.

Duration: Between asanas, 1 or 2 minutes to relax the body. For relaxation, depending to time availability.

Awareness: Physical – first to relax the body in comfortable positioning and then on breathing. Spiritual – on solar plexus (manipura) chakra or sacral (swadhisthana) chakra.

Benefits: Opens the hips and the pelvic floor region and removes congestion. Creates more space in the abdomen area. With the hands extension backwards can help open up the chest and stretch the shoulder blades. Stretches the adductors and groin area. It is a relaxing, calming and energizing practice. Can work as preparatory asana for squatting poses.

Precautions: If the supine positioning feels uncomfortable or gives dizziness, avoid practice.

Note: It is strongly recommended to practice during the third trimester.

35. Happy Baby Pose – Ananda Balasana

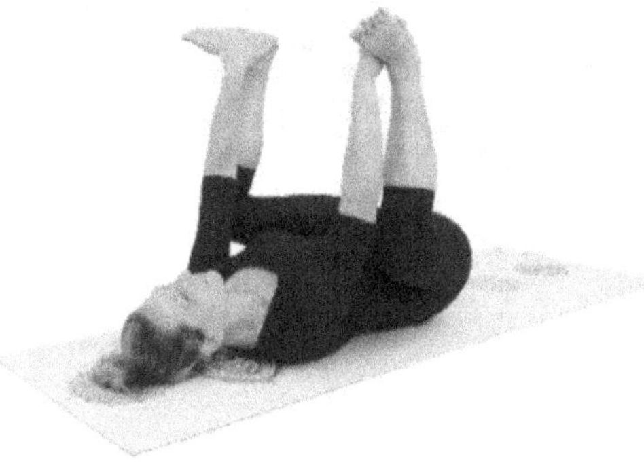

Practice: Lie on the back with the knees bent on the ground. The head and shoulders should remain on the ground through the practice. Slowly bring one leg at a time closer to the chest area and grasp the soles of the feet from the inside or outside, whichever feels more comfortable. The knees should be facing towards the armpits and be spread apart. This is the starting position. Can remain at this position with normal breathing for 15-20 easy counts.

Variation: From starting position and with the heels flexed into the hands, rock to a gentle side to side for 15-20 times to massage the spinal cord and the lower back. This variation should be practiced with ease, no strain and complete balance during the pregnancy.

Breathing: Normal breathing.

Awareness: Physical – on breathing and stretching the lower back, spine and gluteal muscles. Spiritual – on sacral (swadhisthana) chakra or root (mooladhara) chakra.

Benefits: Stretches and releases tension in the back region, spinal column and gluteal muscles. Stretches and flexes the inner thighs, hamstrings, groin and hips. Help on stress and anxiety management, lowers heart rate and releases fatigue.

Precautions: Those with neck or knee injuries should avoid this practice. During pregnancy, especially from second trimester onwards, would-be-mum should have the head and upper back in inclined position with the support of cushions or a bolster.

Note: Can be incorporated in the beginning, middle or end of class as a relaxation and stretching asana. If practitioner cannot keep shoulders flat on the ground during practice, can hold on the ankles or shins. If head is not comfortably flat on the mat, should use a cushion or a rolled blanker as a support system underneath the neck during the first and fourth trimester.

36. Extended Supine Hand to Big Toe Pose – Utthita Supta Padangusthasana

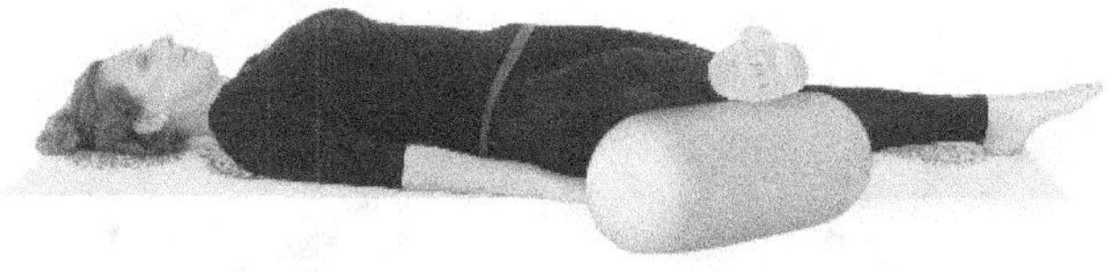

Practice: Have to the side of the right knee or thigh a strong bolster or yoga block and come to a supine position. The hands could be on the side of the torso or could position the palms under the buttocks to help the leg raise and extension without any jerk movement. Inhale to raise the right leg and continuously exhale to extend it to the side and rest it on top of the bolster. Stay in that position for 5-10 normal breaths. Slowly release the extended leg and gently return to original position. Repeat the same with the left leg.

Breathing: Inhale to raise the leg. Exhale to extend and rest the leg on the bolster. Normal breathing at the final position.

Awareness: Physical – on breathing and stretching gently the extended leg without any jerk movement on the leg lift and extension. Spiritual – on root (mooladhara) chakra or sacral (swadhisthana) chakra.

Benefits: Relieves from lower back pain and balances the two sides of the back with the asymmetric positioning. Relieves from arthritis pain in the hips and knees. Aligns the pelvis. The extended leg to the side help stretch the calves, inner thighs, hamstrings, groins and adductors without putting any extra pressure on the vertebrae.

Precautions: In case of overstretch can tear the hamstring muscles. Limit of the position is until the point there is no core engagement and breathing is normal with no strain. Those with high blood pressure and severe spinal conditions should avoid practice. From mid second trimester should add a folded blanket under the head as a precaution. Not to be practiced on third trimester.

37. Legs Up The Wall Pose – Viparita Karani

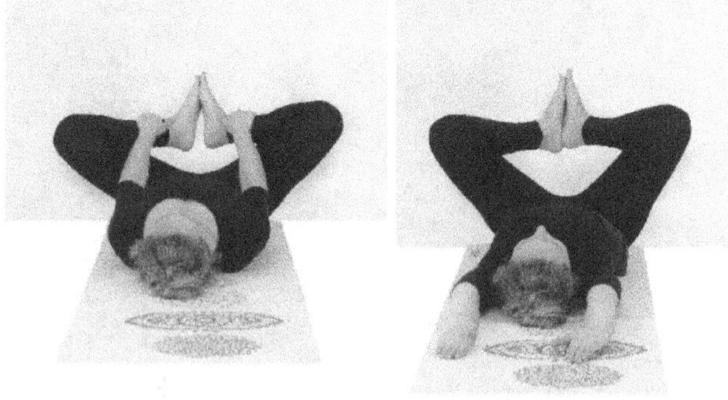

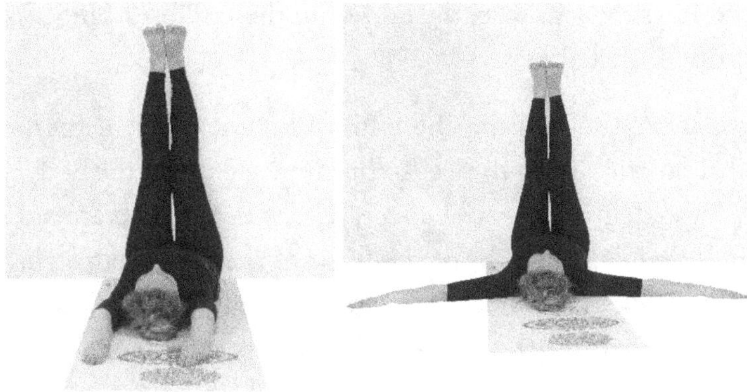

Practice: The Legs up the wall is a variation of Upside-Down Seal (Viparita Karani) and is a gentle restorative asana. Props such as soft pillows or cushions and folded blanket should be close by to support body when needed, especially from second trimester onwards. Position near a wall in Base Position where the left side of the body is touching the wall. Inhale, Exhale and lie on the back and gently move the legs up to the wall with soles of the feet facing upwards. Feet should be comfortably wide apart so there is no squeeze effect to hold them, so there is no pressure on the belly. Alternatively, to increase the stretch, bend the knees and touch the soles together. Then, slide the outer edges of the feet down and bring the heels closer to pelvic floor. Adjust the body to a comfortable position, by moving the buttocks away from the wall especially after second trimester. The back and the head to rest on the ground. With the use of the hands supporting the hips, lift hips up to slide a soft pillow or a folded blanket to lower the curve of the lower back for maximum comfort. If support with a prop is needed between the back of the head and the ground, tilt head up and slide the prop at this stage. The head and the neck should be in neutral position, facing up the ceiling, the throat and the face to be softened. Close the eyes and breath normally or practice a pranayama technique. Should hold the position for at least 5 minutes or longer. When ready to release the pose, exhale and roll to any one side. Inhale to sit up.

Breathing: Normal breathing

Duration: 5 to 10 minutes

Awareness: Physical – to relax the body and then on breathing. Spiritual – throat (vishuddhi) chakra.

Benefits: Can sooth and calm the mind. Promotes the energy movement and blood circulation from the legs to the upper center of the body. Prevents varicose veins, edema and swollen feet, relaxes tired and cramped feet and the pelvic floor. Great stretch for the front of the torso, hamstrings, lower back and the back of the neck. Strengthens capillary circulation of facial muscles and the skin of the face to look younger. Promotes relaxation to the heart. Increases metabolism in body cells which results in fat reduction around the waist. Therapeutic benefits: relieving the nervous system and reducing stress, anxiety, insomnia, help on headache, migraine, arthritis, digestive disorders and stimulates blood pressure. The longer the duration of practice, the best results achieved for a rejuvenated self.

Precautions: It is a mild inversion asana, and if woman is still on lochia or during menstruation should avoid practice. Women with glaucoma or other severe eye conditions should also avoid this asana. Those with serious back and neck issues should practice only in the presence of a certified yoga teacher. As a precaution, if during practice a tingling in the feet is experienced, should bend the knees and touch the soles and bring the heels closer to the pelvic floor.

Meditation Asanas

The aim of the meditation asanas is to sit comfortably for long duration without moving the body. The spine should be naturally erect. When practicing deep meditation, these practices are recommended as it is essential to remain awake and alert of the surroundings. Can prepare the physical body for sitting in any of the meditation asanas for long duration with practices from Pawanmuktasana series. Can prepare the mind for sitting in stillness with affirmations such as: "I am steady as a rock". To achieve comfort and stillness can use a small cushion of a doughnut type under the buttocks.

If there is discomfort or pain in the legs during practice, slowly release the pose and massage the legs. As soon as the blood flow returns to normal levels, there should no longer be any discomfort; at this point can resume practice. Practitioner must be aware of the knees while coming in and out of these poses in order not to strain them.

Practice 2-3 rounds of meditation asanas at equal time per leg. The legs should be alternated so balance is maintained on both sides of the body.

38. Easy Pose – Sukhasana

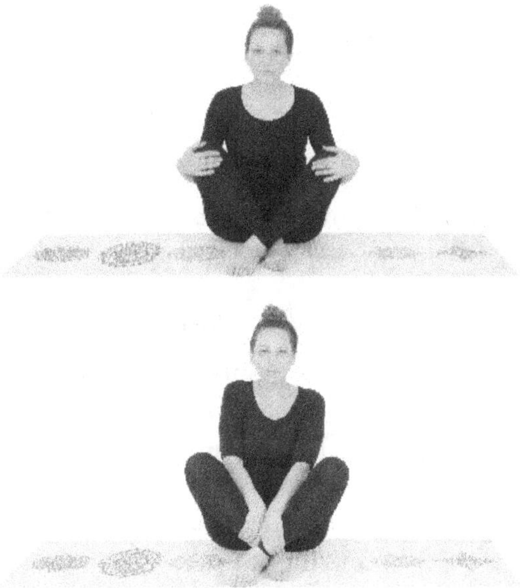

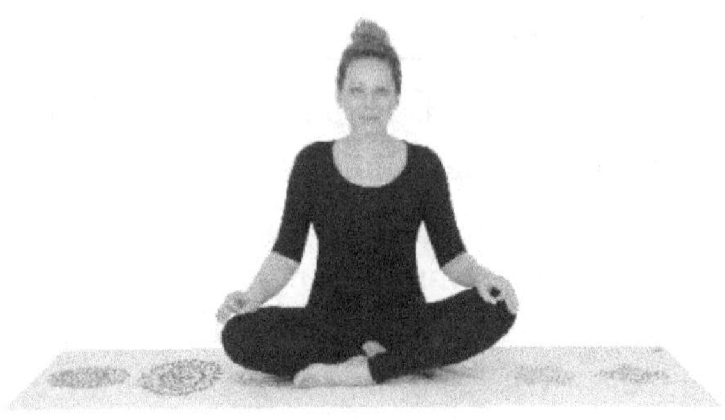

Practice: Bend the knees close to perineum and cross over the soles of the feet. With the help of the hands lower the knees aiming the knees to touch the ground and position both feet under their opposite thigh. Alternatively, with the legs straightened in front of the body, bend one leg and position the foot under the opposite thigh. Bend the other leg and also position the foot under the opposite thigh. Sitting should be on the sit bones. The head, neck and spine should be comfortably upright and aligned. Can relax the hands on the knees in Chin or Jnana Mudra. Close the eyes.

During the 2nd trimester the heels should be slightly away from the groin, when on third trimester should be further away. Use of props such as cushions or yoga blocks to support knees if needed.

Breathing: Normal breathing or practice pranayama techniques.

Duration: Depending the practice and time availability. Can be adopted during meditation practices.

Awareness: Physical; on breathing and loosen the body and relax the eyes completely. Spiritual – on crown (sahasrara) chakra.

Benefits: It is the easiest and most comfortable meditative posture of all. It is recommended to adopt Sukhasana during a pregnancy, especially if practitioner is not experienced with the other meditation postures. It enhances mental and physical balance without causing any pain or ill effect to all practitioners.

39. Half Lotus Pose – Ardha Padmasana

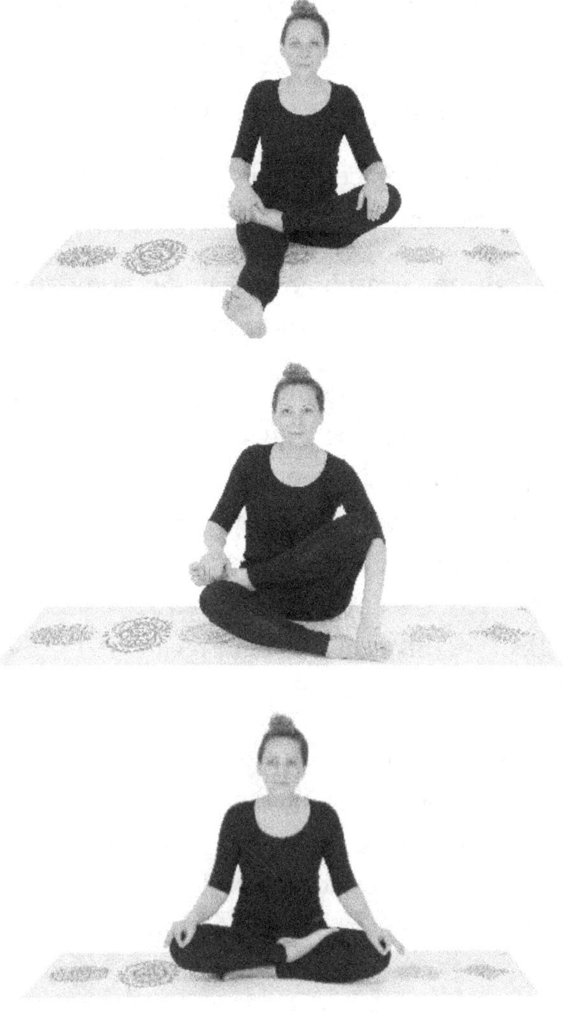

Practice: Similar to Sukhasana, bend the knees close to perineum and cross over the soles of the feet. With the help of the hands lower the knees aiming the knees to touch the ground and position one foot on the inside of the opposite thigh and the other foot on top of the opposite thigh. Alternatively, with the legs straightened in front of the body, bend one leg and position lone foot on the inside of pade opposite thigh and the other foot on top of the opposite thigh. The upper heel should be as near as possible to the groin area. Adjust position to be comfortable and without any strain, sitting comfortably with the legs as the firm sitting foundation. The head, neck and spine should be comfortably upright and aligned. Can relax the hands on the knees in Jnana Mudra. Close the eyes.

Breathing: Normal breathing or practice pranayama techniques.

Duration: Depending the practice and time availability. Can be adopted during meditation practices.

Awareness: Physical; on breathing, loosen the body and relax the eyes completely. Spiritual; Can activate and balance all chakras.

Benefits: Can be adopted during pregnancy, however it is recommended to adopt Sukhasana during that time, especially if practitioner is not experienced in yoga. It allows the body to be held still for longer time, while the legs are the firm sitting foundation and the trunk and head keep steady. When the body is steady, the mind calms and quietens the thoughts, the breath slows down, reduces any muscular tension and can help lowering blood pressure. Because this asana applies pressure to the sacrum, can relax the nervous system.

Precautions: If suffering from sciatica or weak or injured knees it is advisable not to perform this asana, but Sukhasana. During pregnancy should not stay too long in that position, as the blood circulation is redirected from the legs to the abdominal area and blood flow to the legs is reduced; however, in that position the digestive system gets stimulated.

40. Hero's Meditation Pose – Dhyana Veerasana

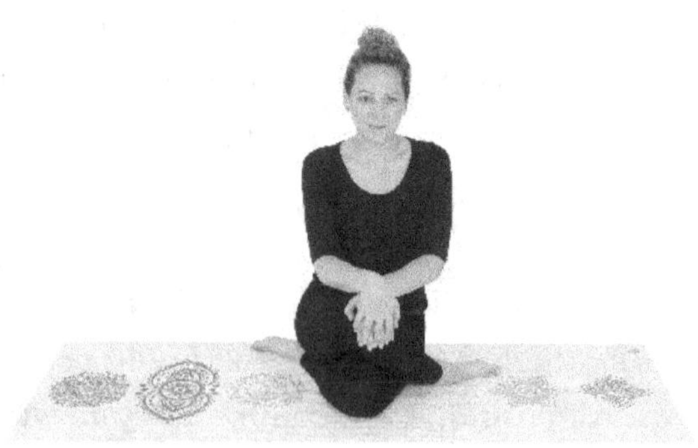

Practice: With the legs straightened in front of the body, bend one leg and position the heel underneath the opposite buttock. Bring the other leg over the top of the bent leg and attempt to touch the opposite buttock. The knees should be aligned one on top of the other. The hands should be comfortably positioned on the feet. The head, neck and spine should be aligned. Close the eyes, relax the whole body.

Breathing: Normal breathing or practice pranayama techniques.

Duration: Depending the practice and time availability. Can be adopted during meditation practices.

Awareness: Physical – on breathing with awareness at the nosetip, and loosening the body and relaxing the eyes completely. Spiritual – on sacral (swadhisthana) chakra or root (mooladhara) chakra.

Benefits: Can be adopted during pregnancy, as it is considered easy and comfortable to sustain for longer duration, since the legs and buttocks are in contact with the floor. By keeping the knees aligned and to the center of the body, the reproductive organs and pelvic is getting massaged and toned up. On this position the outer muscles of the thigh are getting stretched.

Precautions: Should avoid practicing if there is a knee or ankle injury. Also, if there are conditions in the thigh, ankle, lower limb, lumbar, neck, joint pain, headache or spinal disorders.

Vajrasana Group of Asanas

Vajrasana is considered to be a meditation asana. Vajra, the major nadi, is directly connected with the genito-urinary system, which is implicitly connected to the sexual energy in the physical body. Therefore, it is advised to be practiced in the pre-conception phase, to also stimulate the reproductive and digestive organs.

In order to practice these asanas for longer duration in time, the knees and ankles must be adequately flexible. Practitioners with weak knees, inflammatory conditions, arthritis, osteoarthritis should avoid practicing.

41. Thunderbolt Pose – Vajrasana/ Virasana

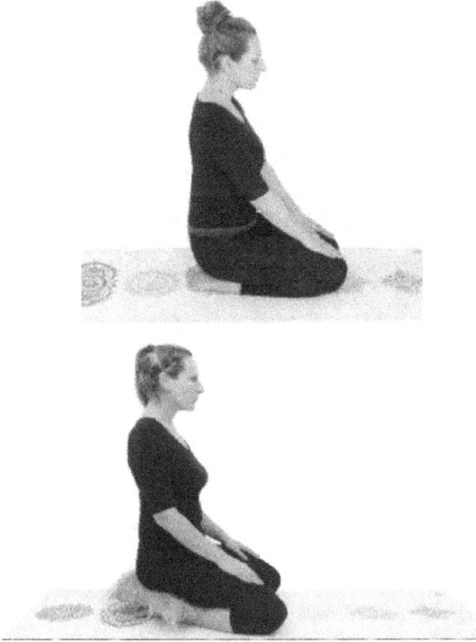

Practice: Kneel with the knees close together during the first and fourth trimester and further apart during the second and third trimester, bring the toes together with heels separated, and lower the buttocks to sit directly on the heels. The palms of the hands to be placed on the knees. Head to be aligned with the spine erect. Relax the whole body with eyes closed and breathe normally.

Modification: If practitioner is not feeling comfortable sitting on vajrasana, then with the support of the hands and knees, carefully lift up the buttocks to slide under a cushion and rest the perineum on top of that. The knees can be wide open to sit comfortably. If need to sit higher to support a better length on the perineum, can use two cushions to sit on.

Virasana: The only difference lies on sitting between the feet with toes pointing outwards. Because of the different elevation here, the perineum is directly rested on the cushion, which has a natural mula bandha3F[4] effect. Impacts greatly on the mental and emotional aspect of the exercise. Creates better balance, stability, grounding and calming effect.

Breathing: Normal breathing through the nostrils.

Awareness: Physical – in the beginning of the practice, practitioners should be aware on the physical sensation and breathing and relaxation has been achieved should focus on the eyebrow center. Spiritual – center of eyebrows, on ajna chakra.

Duration: Depending on time availability and class planning.

Benefits: It is the only practice that can be done right after a meal because it helps on digestive system conditions, such as constipation, indigestion, acidity. Strengthens the pelvic muscles. Prevents hernia and relieves hemorrhoids. Straighten naturally the spinal column. Those who suffer from lumbar pain or hip joint pain can sit on this position when practicing instead of any other seated asana. Helps the blood flow and supply in the belly region and the placenta. Because it stimulates the vajra nadi4F[5], life force energy is increased in sushumna5F[6], therefore increases the oxygen flow particularly in the chest area.

---

[4] A Sanskrit term for *root locked*, a natural way to draw in and up the root (mooladhara) chakra.

[5] Vajra Nadi is one of the channels through which prana or else life force energy travels in the human body. Vajra in Sanskrit means thunderbolt and Nadi means channel.

[6] Sushumna Nadi is one of the three main nadis, where the other two are ida and pingala. Sushumna Nadi is the central channel that connects all seven chakras.

Precautions: Those with knee or ankle conditions should not sit on this position. Those who experience pain in the thighs during practice, but they don't have any knee or ankle conditions, could separate the knees slightly without adjusting the position.

Note: First trimester, try to bring the knees closer together. second trimester, keep the knees slightly separated to accommodate nicely the belly. third trimester, is not advisable to practice, as the gained weight can overload the knee joints; however, if practiced, the use of a cushion is mandatory. The use of a cushion is highly recommended during pregnancy practice, because in this asana one can sit for longer periods of time, and the cushion will take tension from the knees. Also, if the perineum is not elevated or not comfortably seated directly on the mat or on a cushion, the quadriceps get internally rotated which will have a wrong ligament pain6F[7] arising. As long as the practitioner is seated comfortably with or without a cushion, there is no problem.

42. Gracious Pose – Bhadrasana

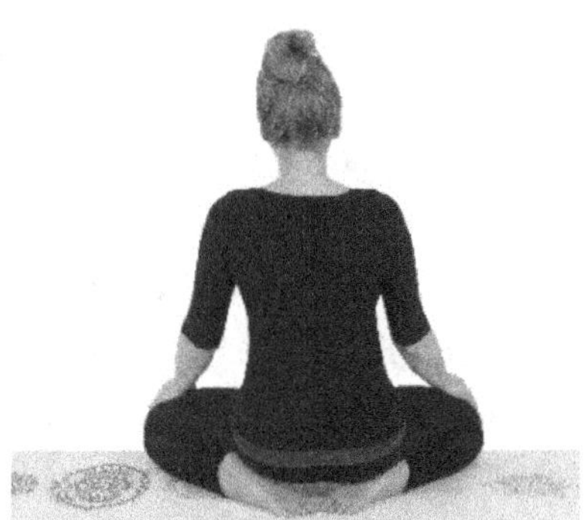

Practice: From Vajrasana, separate the knees wide open and comfortably allow the buttocks and perineum to sit flat and keep the toes in contact with the ground. Place the palms on the knees facing down. With normal breathing, focus on the nosetip with the eyes open. Close the eyes when they get tired for 10-20 seconds, open the eyes and repeat the practice.

---

[7] The ligaments are connected from the belly to the pubic bone and when there is an extreme stretch practitioner may experience some pain later on.

Breathing: Normal breathing.

Awareness: Physical – on breathing; can also practice Kegel exercises on that pose. Spiritual – on root (mooladhara) chakra.

Precautions: Those with knees, hips or groin conditions should avoid practice. If gazing at the nosetip brings nausea or dizziness, avoid gazing and practice only kegels or meditation on this pose.

Note: If unable to sit flat on the ground the buttocks and perineum, a folded blanket must be used as a support system under the buttocks to activate root chakra.

43. Cow's Face Pose – Gomukhasana

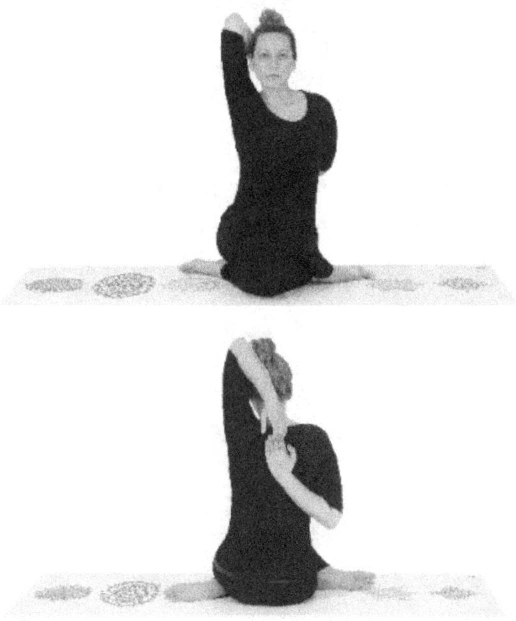

Practice: This practice is performed while on Dhyana Veerasana. During the first trimester only, it could be performed, however, from second trimester onwards it is advisable to separate the crossing of both limbs together and modify the practice by sitting on Vajrasana. Start with the palms of the hands on the knees. Inhale to raise one hand and bend it over the opposite shoulder. Stretch the other hand to the side and bend it behind the back, where the back of the hand should touch the spine while the opposite palm of the hand rests in the spine. Attempt to touch the fingers of both hands behind the back. The raised elbow should be positioned behind the ear so that the head is resting on the inside of the raised arm. The head should be slightly back and the spine erect. Inhale to release the hand. Repeat the same with the other hand to complete 1 round. Can practice 3-5 rounds.

Modification 1:

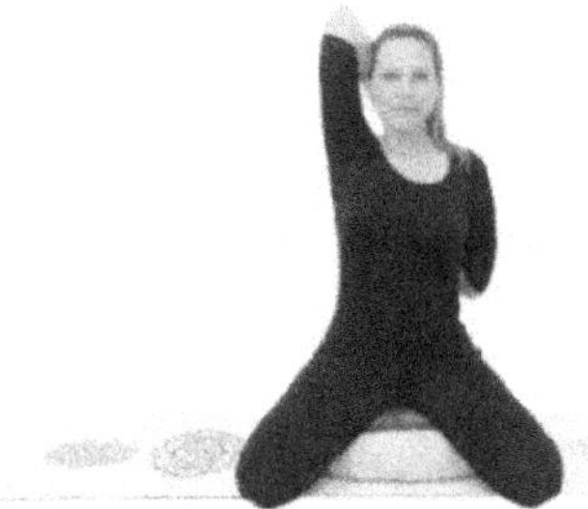

To support comfortable positioning, or for those who can't sit directly on Vajrasana or Virasana, can use the support of a cushion to sit on to elevate the perineum.

Modification 2:

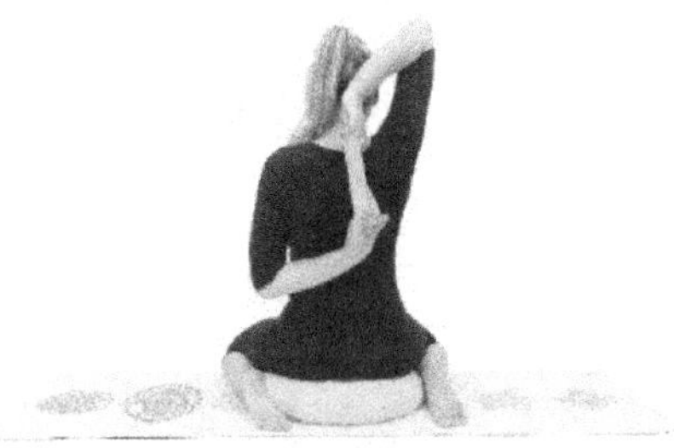

If cannot touch the fingers of both hands, can use a thera-band or a cloth to hold the final position. Aim of this modified asana is to open up the chest and by positioning the head slightly back you achieve maximum stretch on the spine.

Breathing: Normal breathing.

Awareness: Physical – on normal breathing and chest opening. Spiritual – on third eye (ajna chakra) or heart (anahata) chakra.

Duration: Maintain the position for 5 breaths.

Benefits: Same as Dhyana Veerasana, and Vajrasana/ Virasana, depending which starting position is used. Especially from fourth trimester onwards for nursing mums, the hands positioning on the final posture are working as chest opener. Can relieve from backache, neck and shoulders stiffness, fatigue, tension, anxiety and improve body posture.

Precautions: Same as Vajrasana or Virasana.

Note: First trimester, try to keep the knees together. second and third trimester, keep the knees separate to accommodate the growing belly. Fourth trimester can practice seated in Dhyana Veerasana.

44. Lion Pose – Simhasana

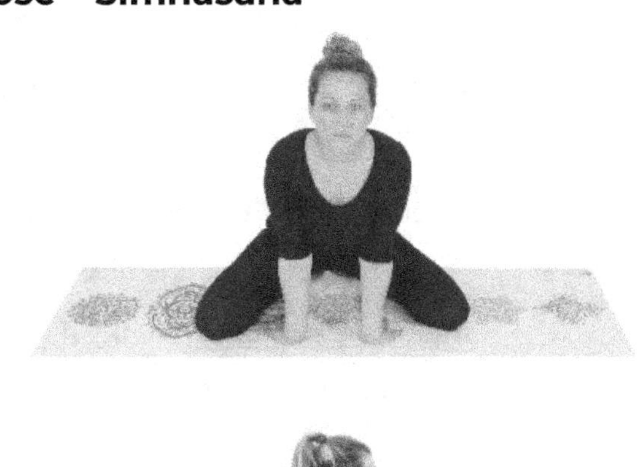

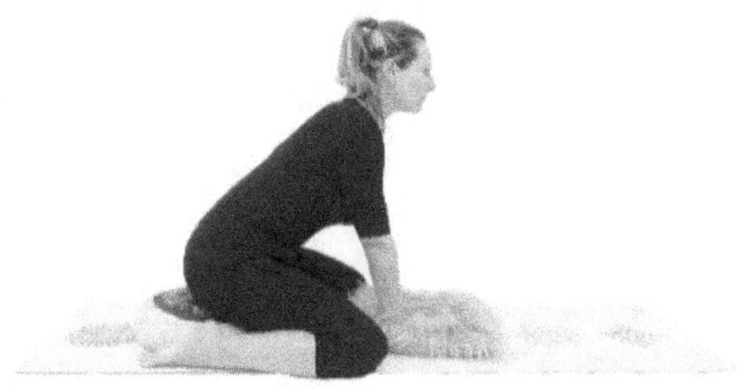

Practice: Sit in Vajrasana without forcing the toes to touch each other. Bring the palms to the ground and between the knees, with the fingers pointing towards the body. Make sure there is a big gap between the belly and the position. It is ideal for maximum practice benefits to have the whole palm on the ground with the meridian points pressed. If this creates discomfort, can use the support of a cushion to place the palms on top of it and give the height needed. The arms and the back should be straight. With the eyes and mouth closed, inhale to bring the chin to the chest and slowly exhale to raise the head slightly backwards to comfortably compress the neck. At this position, put the awareness and inner gaze at the eyebrow center, performing the shambhavi mudra. If practitioner still suffers from nausea and dizziness can also practice with the eyes open by fixing the gaze at a point on the ceiling.

Breathing: Normal breathing. Synchronize inhalation to bring chin to the chest and on exhalation to raise the head up.

Duration: Stay in the final position for 3-5 normal breaths and return to the center. Repeat 5-10 rounds daily to maintain good health.

Awareness: Physical – on keeping the arms and back straight. Spiritual – on third eye (ajna) chakra or throat (vishuddhi) chakra.

Benefits: Stretches the spinal cord, helps to correct body posture, opens the chest and offers total stability for the physical body.

Precautions: Those with wrist injuries should avoid the practice. Those with knees or hips injuries could practice seated on a chair.

Note: This is a sitting quietly asana related to the waiting lion for some action. In yogic and tantric scriptures, the practice of shambhavi mudra is used to enter deep meditative states, for which the mind needs to be balanced to experience consciousness at higher levels.

45. Roaring Lion Pose – Simhagarjanasana

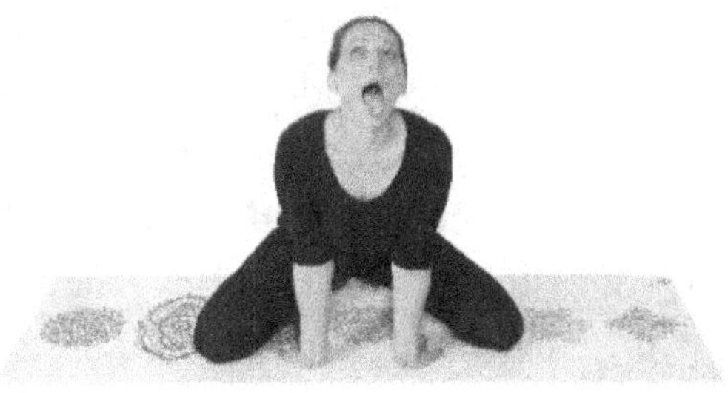

Practice: Sit in Simhasana. With the eyes open, practice the shambhavi mudra to gaze at the eyebrow center. The whole body should be relaxed. Should maintain normal breathing until this point. Inhale slowly through the nostrils, open the mouth widely to extend the tongue as far out as possible, and exhale slowly through the mouth by making the sound of "aaa" from the throat. The sound must be coming out naturally without any force. At the end of exhalation, close the mouth and continue normal breathing. This is 1 round. From the next round, try to adopt the shambhavi mudra.

Variation: During the production of the sound, can move the tongue left and right and/or up and down.

Breathing: Normal breathing to sit in simhasana. Slow and deep inhalation through the nose before slow exhalation from the mouth.

Duration: Can practice 5-10 rounds daily and at any convenient time. Between each round can take a break for 2-3 slow breaths through the nostrils to relax the eyes, tongue and mouth.

Awareness: Physical – on keeping the arms and back straight and the awareness in the eyes and tongue. On inhalation, focus on the breath. On exhalation focus on the "aaa" sound produced, the release of emotions and the throat area. Spiritual – on third eye (ajna) chakra or throat (vishuddhi) chakra.

Benefits: Parts benefited from this asanas are the face, eyes, ears, nose, mouth, tongue, vocal chords, throat, chest, respiratory tract, diaphragm, abdomen, hands and fingers. Relaxes the facial muscles and helps reduce stress and tension on the face and its parts. Helps on bleary or burning eyes, delays aging by helping remove wrinkles. Stimulates the throat muscles and helps to keep them firm as we continue to age. Can cure stuttering, teeth grinding, clenched jaws, helps get rid of bad breath, and exercise the tongue with its full stretch outside the mouth. Relaxes the neck muscles and relieves back pain. Helps reduce stress and tension on the chest and diaphragm, get rid of any respiratory tract infections. Enhances memory and poor concentration we get thought a pregnancy. Those who use their voice as a profession, can be helped to improve the voice tone and texture.

Precautions: Those with wrist injuries should avoid the practice. Those with knees or hips injuries could practice seated on a chair.

Note: Those who find it difficult to adopt the shambhavi mudra can close their eyes or gaze up towards the ceiling. Not to be practiced after the first trimester as the extra weight gained can aggravate the knee joints.

46. Child's Pose – Shashankasana

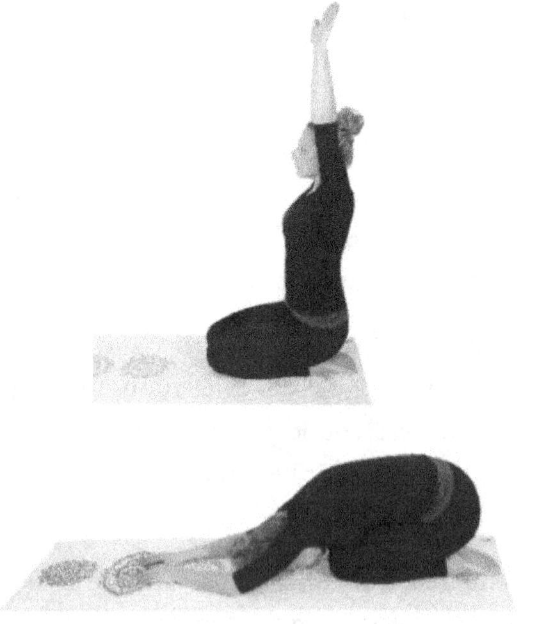

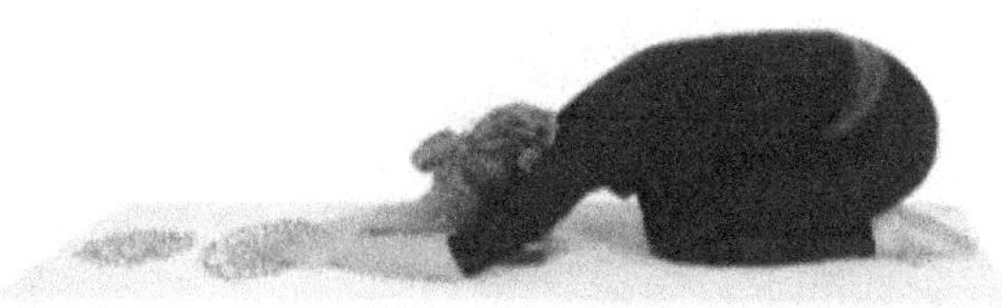

Practice: During the pre-conception, first trimester and fourth trimester, can practice the traditional Shashankasana. Coming to pose, from Vajrasana, inhale to raise the hands up and on exhalation slowly bend the body forward from the hips so the hands and forehead can rest on the ground in front of the knees. Can use one or two cushions or a yoga block to rest the forehead if needed. Relax the forearms slightly bent flat on the ground. When on final position, breath normally through the nostrils for 2 deep and long breaths. To release the pose, inhale and slowly with no jerky movement raise the arms and truck to vajrasana. Exhale to bring the hands to the knees. This is 1 round and can practice 3-5 rounds.

Modification 1: During the first trimester, the initial step of raising the hands up and bending forward may cause dizziness and nausea effect to some women. Instead, can walk down the floor with the palms of the hands and bring gently the body to final position. To release the pose, while exhaling, slowly walk back to vajrasana. Also the use of props to support the rested forehead can reduce nausea effects. This modification can be used at any phase of the four trimesters to tone up the back and pelvic muscles.

Modification 2:

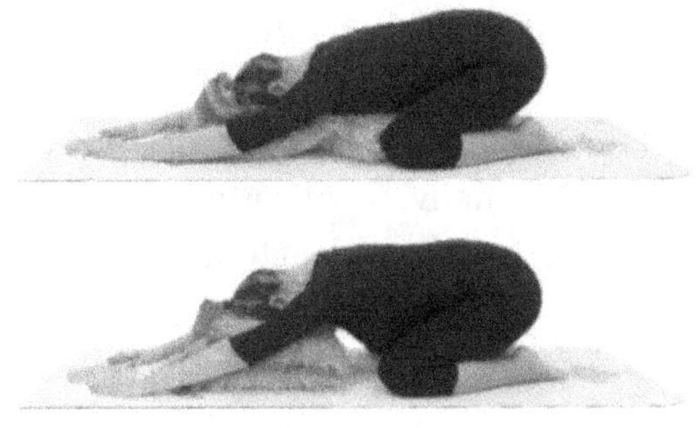

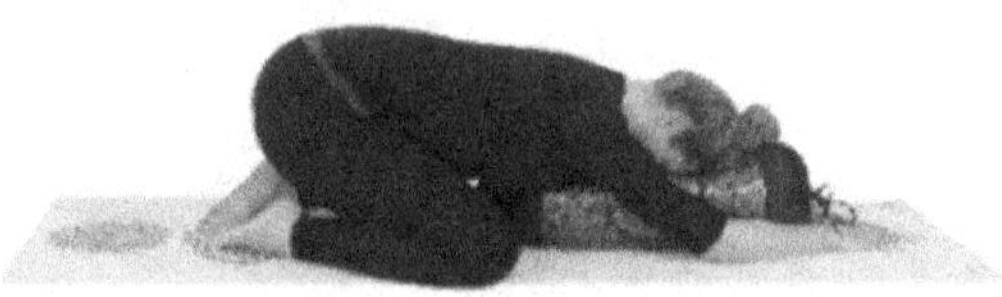

During second and third trimester, should have a good gap between the knees and it is ideal to use a pillow, bolster or cushions to support the head and/or breast. If no support is needed for the breasts, can use one or two cushions to rest the forehead on so the belly is nicely accommodated. As the pregnancy progresses, if a practitioner feels the need to support the growing belly, can add a cushion between the belly and the ground as it may feel comfortable.

Modification 3:

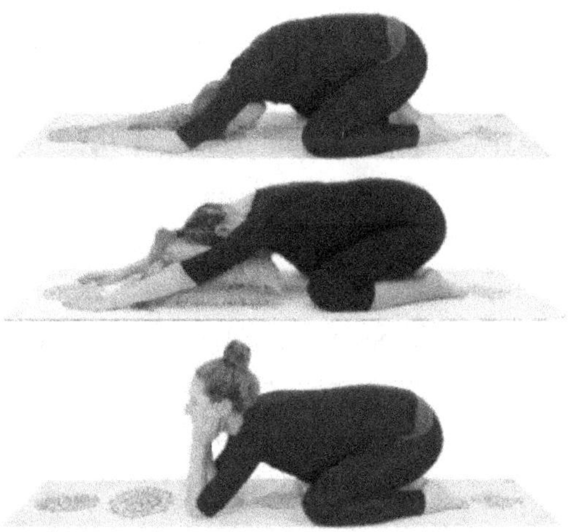

During the third trimester, and especially towards the end, the size of the growing belly makes it difficult and uncomfortable to be in the final position with the spine, arms and head straight. In that final position may rest the forehead on the ground with the spine aligned to the floor, similar to table top position. Alternatively, can use props to rest the forehead and the hands should be bent from the elbows in a wider angle. Or, can stretch the back by holding the head from the jaws with the palms of the hands.

Breathing: Inhale to raise hands up. Exhale to bend the body forward. Normal breathing.

Duration: Practice for 3-10 minutes on comfortably holding the final position, according to your level.

Awareness: Physical – on the alignment of the arms, neck and head and on breath synchronization when coming to position and releasing it. Spiritual – on navel (manipura) chakra or pelvic (swadhisthana) chakra.

Benefits: Modification 1 – walking forward with the hands will exert pressure from abdomen area and pelvis. Modification 2 – rested forehead on props can help those with higher blood pressure at any phase in life including during the pregnancy. Modification 3 – it still stretches and strengthens the back muscles and spinal cord, although with lesser effects since the gravity of the belly doesn't allow complete stretching of the spine and arms. Generally, helps opening up the pelvis and hips. Removes tension and pain from the lower back. Helps realign the spine. Creates space around the belly. It is a soothing and energizing asana which relieves nausea. Helps the baby move into anterior position when practicing in the third trimester.

Precautions: Those who suffer from vertigo or nausea, very high blood pressure and back conditions should avoid this asana.

Note: Compression of the belly must be avoided at all times. If there is pain experienced in the knees, should place a cushion or folded blanket under the buttocks.

47. Extended Puppy Pose – Uttana Shishosana

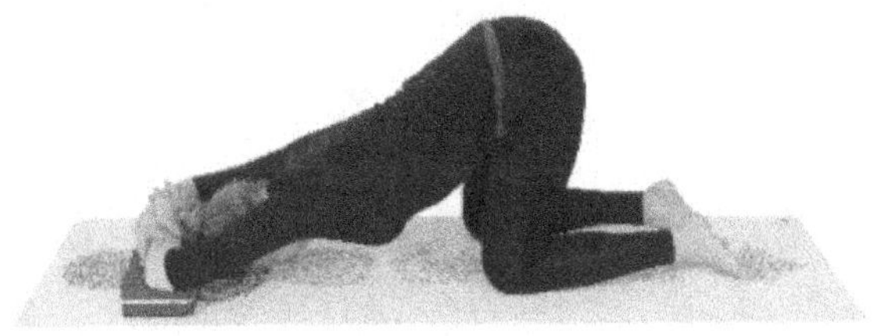

Practice: From Bharmanasana, with the knees apart under the hips, walk down with the hands in front of the body to allow the chest come closer to the ground and the forehead to rest on the ground. During pregnancy, use two yoga blocks to rest the elbows on and help the body to be in a more comfortable alignment and height. Hand lock the arms by grasping opposite elbows. Stay in the position for 5-10 comfortable breaths. To release the pose, unlock the hands, place the palms on the ground, slowly lift up the body and walk towards the body with the hands, until your reach table-top position.

Breathing: Normal breathing.

Duration: 5-10 comfortable breaths.

Awareness: Physical – on breathing and stretching the upper back, spine, arms and shoulders. Spiritual – on heart (anahata) chakra.

Benefits: Stretches the upper back, spine, arms and shoulders. The spinal stretch helps to improve body posture and flow of prana is also increased as it opens the chest activating the lungs and heart. Improves blood circulation. This pose is considered as a restorative one for those suffering from hips and back pains. Can also help on insomnia, as it relaxes the body and mind. During the pregnancy, can also give relief from nausea. If labor is progressing very fast can practice this asana to slow it down.

Precautions: Not to be practiced by those with severe lower back pain, knee or hip injuries; those with stiff arms and shoulders should not overstretch; those with extreme stiffness do not practice. Not to be practiced during the third trimester, as the blood circulates in the opposite direction if performed for a longer duration.

Note: During the practice should not overstretch, should not strain.

48. Sleeping Thunderbolt Pose – Supta Vajrasana

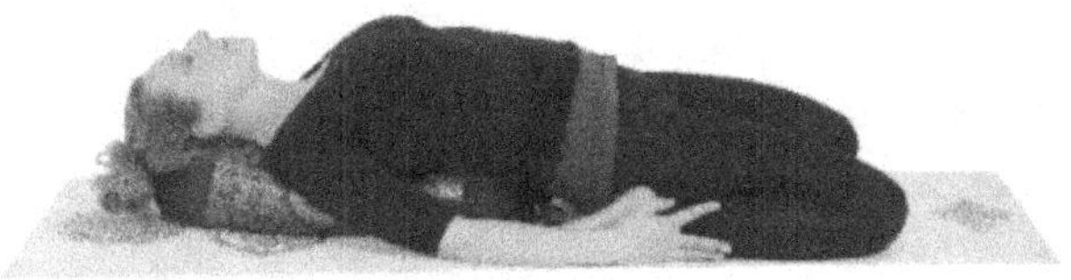

Practice: During pregnancy, should practice only with the support of a bolster positioned across the spine. From Vajrasana bend back with the support of the elbows – one at a time. The body at this stage must be supported on the elbows. Slowly, release the elbows and gently lie the back on the bolster. The hands can be placed either on the thighs, or on the ankles or on the side of the body. The knees should remain in contact with the ground at all times; if not, incline the body higher with a second bolster. Remain at this position with normal breathing for as long as it feels comfortable. There should be no strain during the practice

Breathing: Normal breathing.

Awareness: Physical – on breathing and stretching the ankles, thighs and hips. Spiritual – on root (swadhisthana) chakra.

Benefits: Improves digestive and respiratory systems. Strengthens and stretches the spine and its muscles and nerves. Stretches and massages the quadriceps, ankles and abdomen area organs. Helps in sciatica pain relief and those suffering from high blood pressure. Relaxes and flexes lower limb tendons, ligaments and knee muscles.

Precautions: Those with ankle, knee, hip, back or spinal conditions should avoid this practice or use more than one bolster to increase the upper body inclination. Should not be practiced if suffering from hernia or other intestinal issues.

Note: Should not attempt to bring the crown of the head on the ground nor arch the spine thuring the pregnancy. Should not practice without the support of a bolster or cushions during pregnancy, as inferior vena cava can be compressed, and belly can be overstretched.

Sun Salutation – Surya Namaskar

49. Sun Salutation – Surya Namaskar

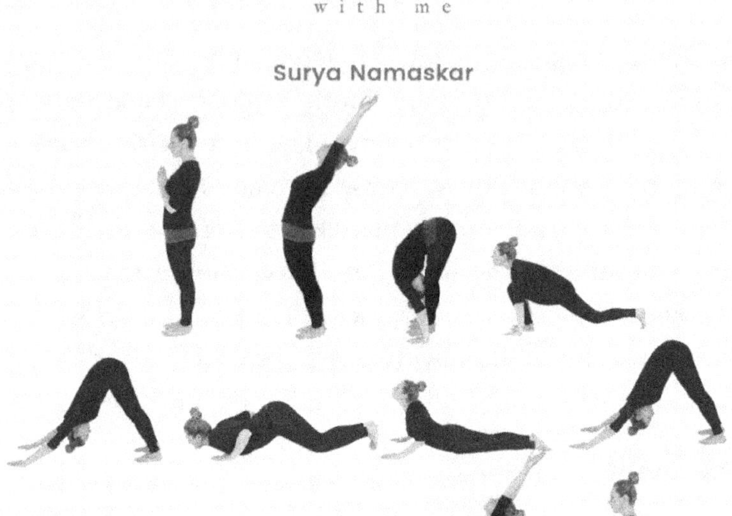

Traditional Sun Salutation can be practiced during pregnancy until the end of first trimester and upon full recovery post childbirth to re-tone up the uterine muscles. However, mothers-to-be who have been advised by their healthcare advisor to bed rest, should not practice Sun Salutation or its variations given in this book. Generally, this is an excellent form of exercise to stimulate and tone up the whole body, as well as boost the emotional well-being. With this group of asanas, the blood circulation is improved, and also strengthens various joints and muscles.

If practitioner feels calm, relaxed and breaths normally, may repeat the traditional or modified Surya Namaskar up to 3-5 times. If at any time during the practice the practitioner feels uncomfortable and strain should stop at once. Practice should not be in the form of cardio, but slow with controlled movements always being aware of safety, allowing room to adjust the body so the belly is never compressed or overstretched.

It can be practiced at any time during the day given the fact the stomach is empty (3-4 hours after last meal). However, *surya* in Sanskrit means *sun* and *namaskar* means *salutations*, therefore, it would be ideal to practice at sunrise, facing east at sunrise, maybe outdoors if conditions allow that. With the eyes closed before commencing practice, connect to breath, ground the body, relax the mind with the breath control, feel harmony within your body, place the awareness to the heart or eyebrow center and visualize the rising sun energizing and infusing your whole body. You may open your eyes and start the practice of Surya Namaskar.

Breathing: Surya Namaskar generates prana the vital energy which activates the psychic body. Therefore, breathing should be steady and rhythmic with the practice of asanas

Awareness: Smoothing the movements. After practice, come to Shavasana to rest and focus on the heartbeat and breathing, as well as the effects on the shoulders, lower back, hips, knees and ankles. Remember, that during second and third trimester Shavasana needs to be modified to an inclined position.

Benefits: If we talk about the anatomy and physiology, all body systems (Skeletal, Muscular, Respiratory, Nervous, Endocrine, Digestive, Reproductive, Cardiovascular and Circulatory) are worked out and stimulated since internal organs are massaged. If we talk about the physical body, it stretches and strengthens the whole body, massages and tones up all the joints, muscles and internal organs, improves flexibility. If we talk about spiritual awareness, the following chakras are activated; sacral (swadhisthana), heart (anahata), throat (vishuddhi) or third-eye (ajna). If practiced daily, Sadhana spiritual practice is complete, as it includes asanas, pranayama, mantra and meditation techniques. In that case, pingala nadi – the pranic life-force channel is regulated which in return balances the energy between mind and body.

Precautions: In the cases of occurrence of fever, acute inflammation, boils or rashes due to toxins released in the body, practice should be stopped and resumed after elimination of these effects. Because the Surya Namaskar is consisted of various poses, each pose should be studied separately for its contra-indication. Nevertheless, if a general rule can be in place, it should not be practiced by those with high blood pressure, heart conditions, have had a stroke, in cases of hernia, intestinal tuberculosis, slipped disc, sciatica, back conditions, knee conditions, ankles conditions and anyone who has been diagnosed with medium or high risk pregnancy.

Precautions: Surya Namaskar has many benefits during pregnancy, and it is always recommended for a self-practitioner to seek professional guidance for correct practicing during pregnancy to maximize its benefits and have a harmless practice for the baby. Practicing on a regular basis is advisable, as random practice may create discomfort during a pregnancy. After completing practice, even during the session, if one feels it is needed, come to Shavasana and relax the whole body by connecting to breath. All asanas should be performed in a gentle and smooth manner, without any force or strain. Every pregnancy is different and before commencing Surya Namaskar, the mother-to-be should consult her healthcare advisor regardless how fit or healthy she may be.

50. Sun Salutation – Surya Namaskar (First Trimester)

Classical Surya Namaskar consists from a group of asanas which are not all practical nor safe as the pregnancy progresses and belly grows. As qualified pre and postnatal yoga teachers, we should be aware of all these asanas we can put together to consist a safe class, create a nice flow for the mum-to-be and be creative! Herein, I give you a modified sun salutation that can be practiced even during the later stages of pregnancy for fit and experienced practitioners.

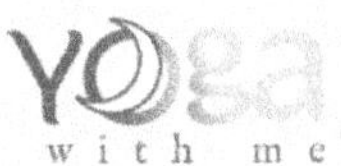

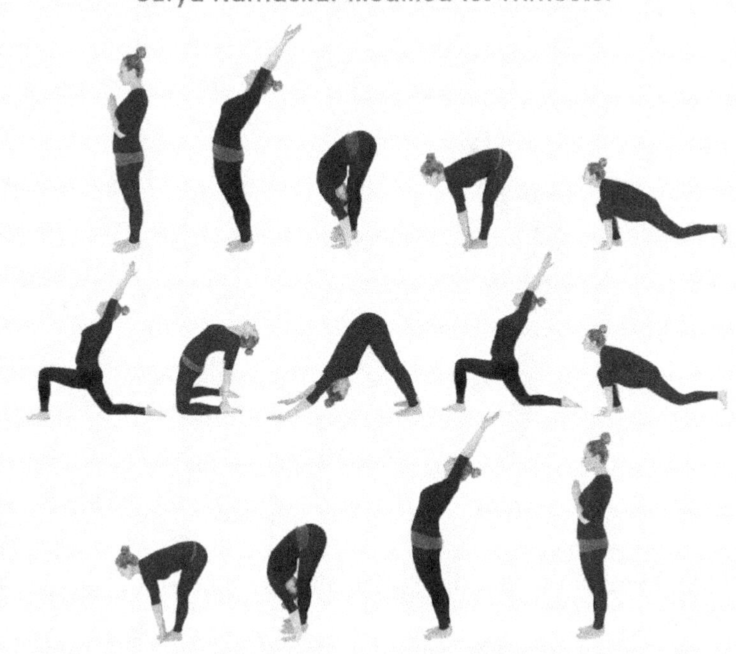

1. From Samasthiti come to Pranamasana with feet placed hip-width or more than that for better balance, especially after second trimester.

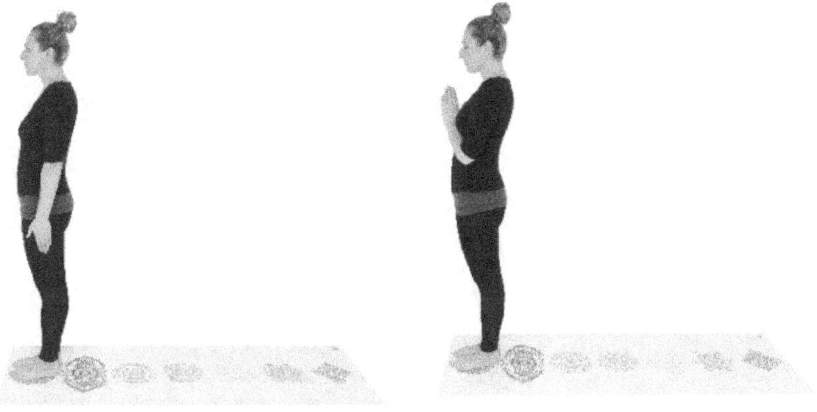

Inhale, raise the arms over the head into Hasta Utthanasana by keeping the spine, head and arms straight. Look at the palms of the hands or in order to avoid dizziness can fix gaze forward to the eyes level.

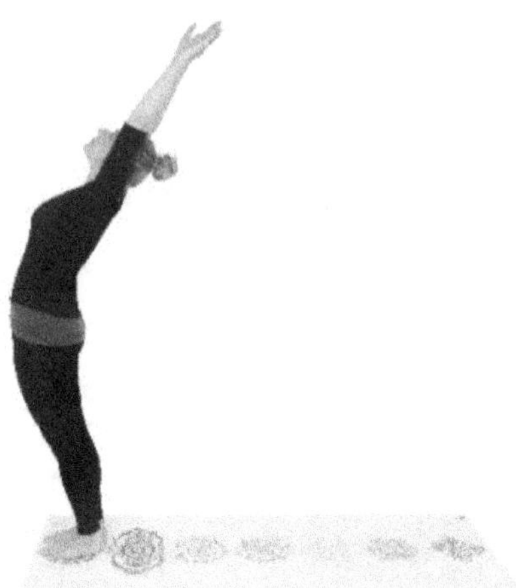

2. Exhale, bend from the hips to Padahastasana.

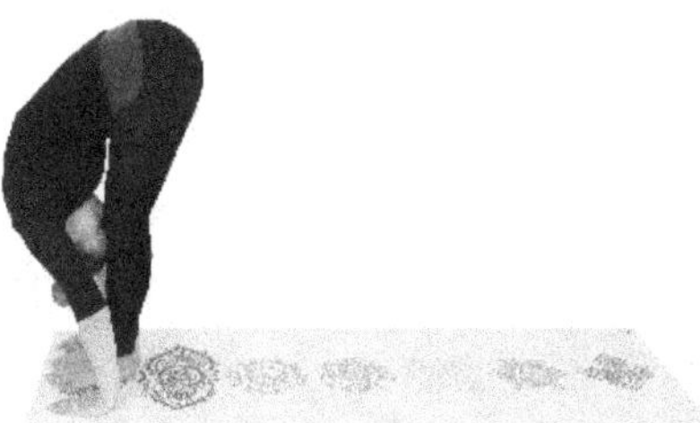

3. Inhale, with the chest forward, fixing the gaze straight and place the hands close to toes or on the shins into Ardha Uttanasana.

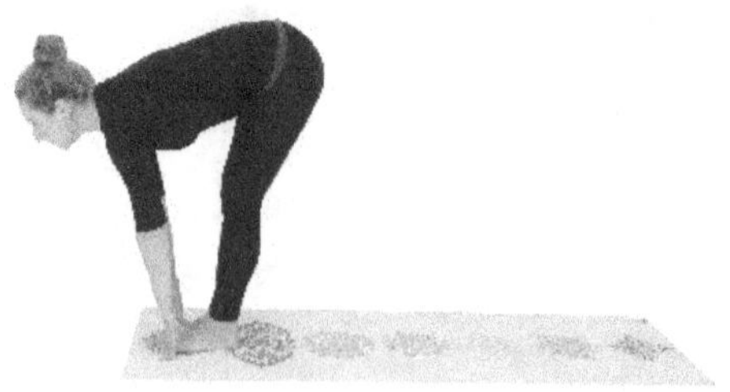

4. Exhale while still looking forward to get into Ashwa Sanchalanasana.

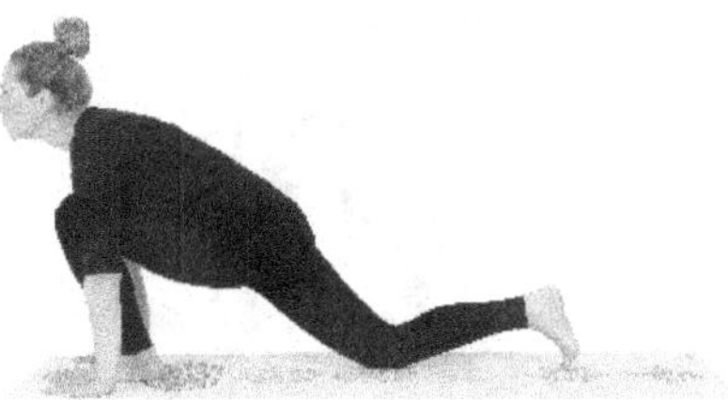

5. Inhale to Ardha Chandrasana.

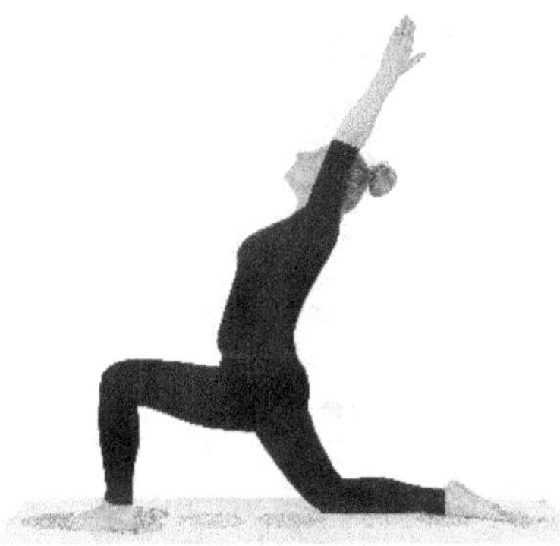

6. Exhale to kneel the other shin. Inhale to arch upper back by taking the hands back into the Ushtrasana or Ardha Ushtrasana.

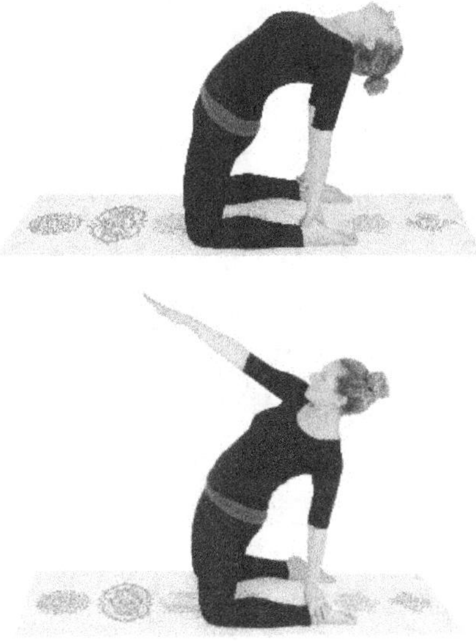

7. Inhale to come to table top position. Exhale, tuck your toes inside and adjust your body to Parvatasana.

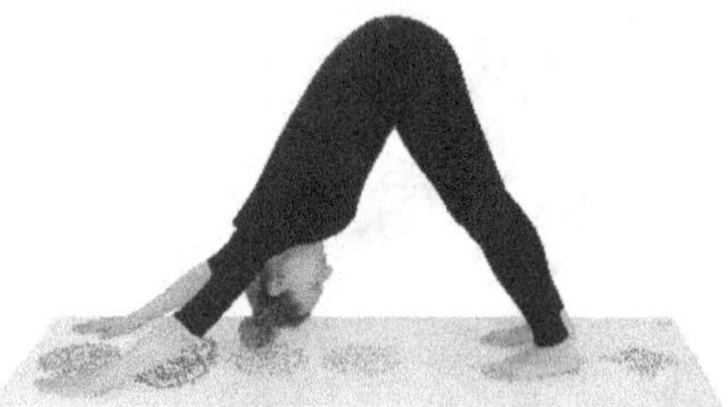

8. Inhale to Ardha Chandrasana.

9. Exhale while still looking forward to get into Ashwa Sanchalanasana.

10. Inhale, with the chest forward, fixing the gaze straight and place the hands on the shins into Ardha Uttanasana.

11. Exhale, bend from the hips to Padahastasana.

12. Inhale, bend your knees a bit and lift yourself up, let your hands reach forward and up to Hasta Utthanasana.

13. Exhale to Pranamasana and then place one hand on the heart and the other on the belly.

51. Sun Salutation – Surya Namaskar (Second & Third Trimester)

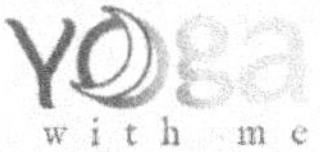

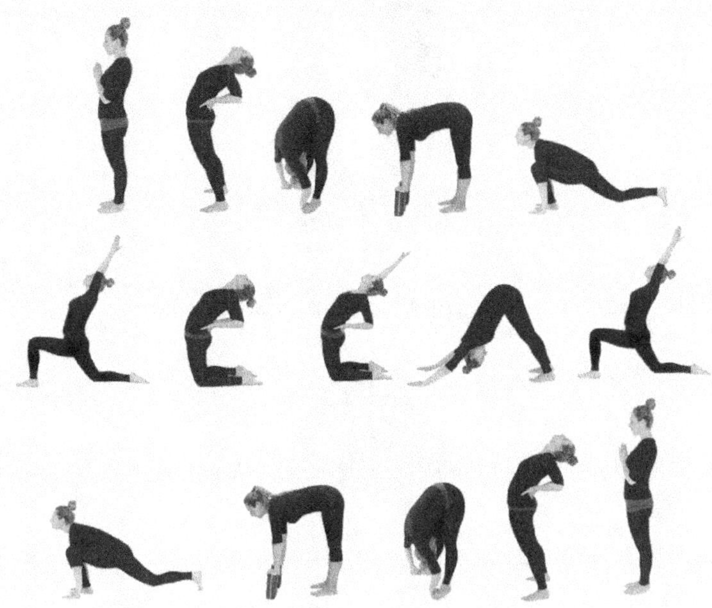

1. From Samasthiti come to Pranamasana with feet placed hip-width or more than that for better balance, as pregnancy is progressing.

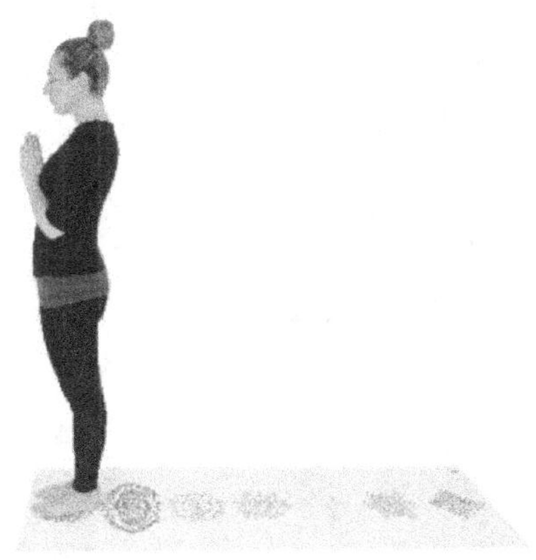

Inhale, to come to a modified Hasta Utthanasana. Instead of raising the arms over the head, can place the palms of the hands on the lumbar area, by maintaining the spine, head aligned.

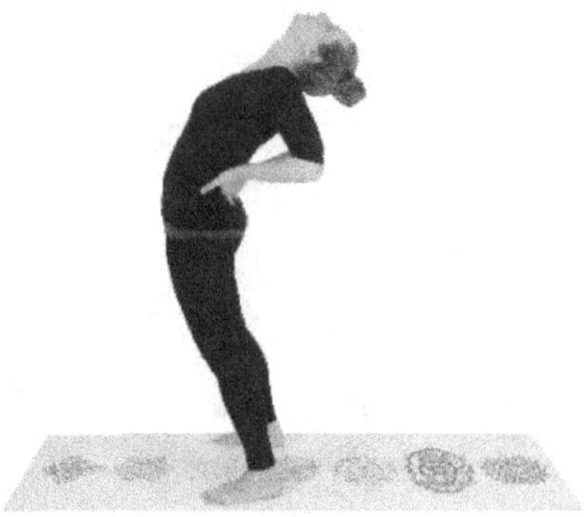

2.   Exhale, bend from the hips to Vayu Nishkasana.

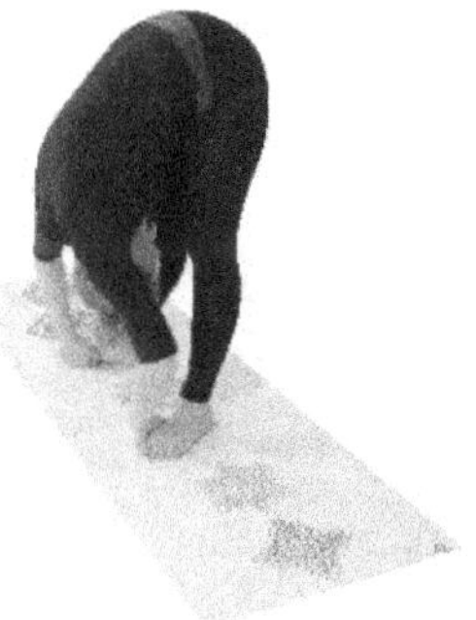

Inhale, into Ardha Uttanasana with the chest forward, fixing the gaze straight and place the hands on the shins during second trimester and during third trimester can use one yoga block per hand to support bent movement and balance.

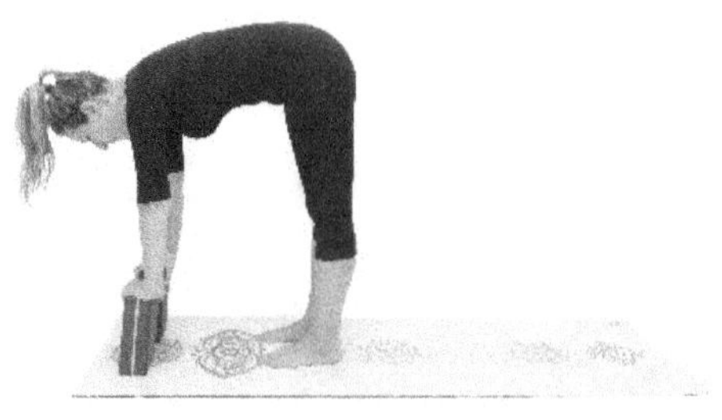

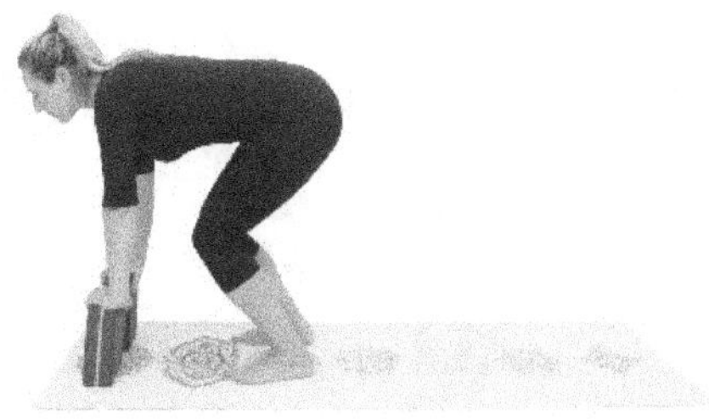

3.   Exhale while still looking forward to get into Ashwa Sanchalanasana.

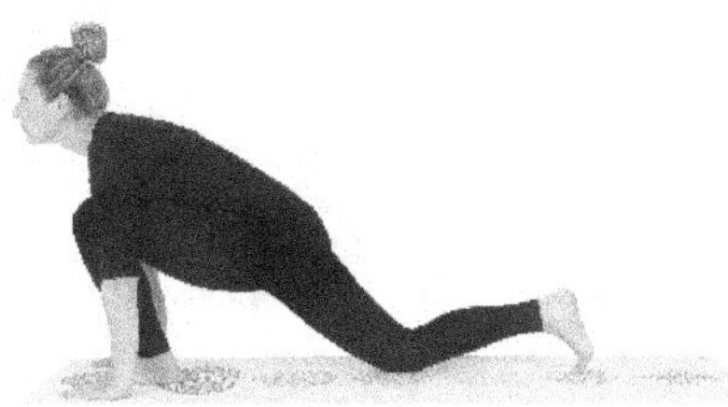

4.   Inhale to Ardha Chandrasana.

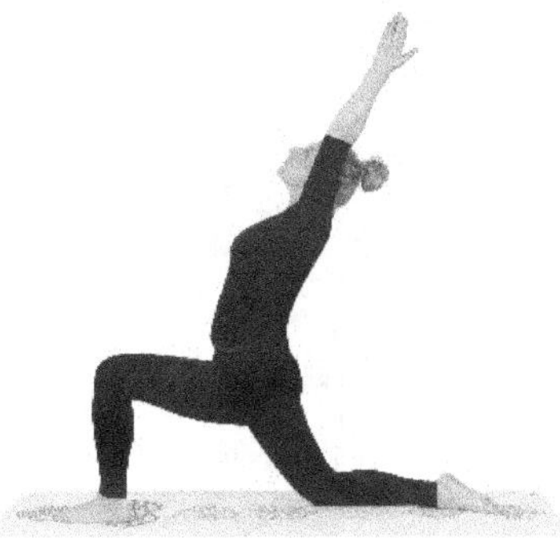

5.   Exhale to kneel the other shin. Inhale to arch upper back by coming into the modified Ushtrasana by positioning the palms of the hands on the lumbar area. Or, can come to Ardha Ushtrasana with one hand touching the same ankle or heel and the opposite hand extended forward in front and higher than the head level by fixing the gaze in the fingers. If strain is experienced by extending the arm forward, practitioner can alternatively extend the arm backwards with the forearm aligned with the head and following the backward bend. The other hand can be positioned with the palm holding the lumbar area.

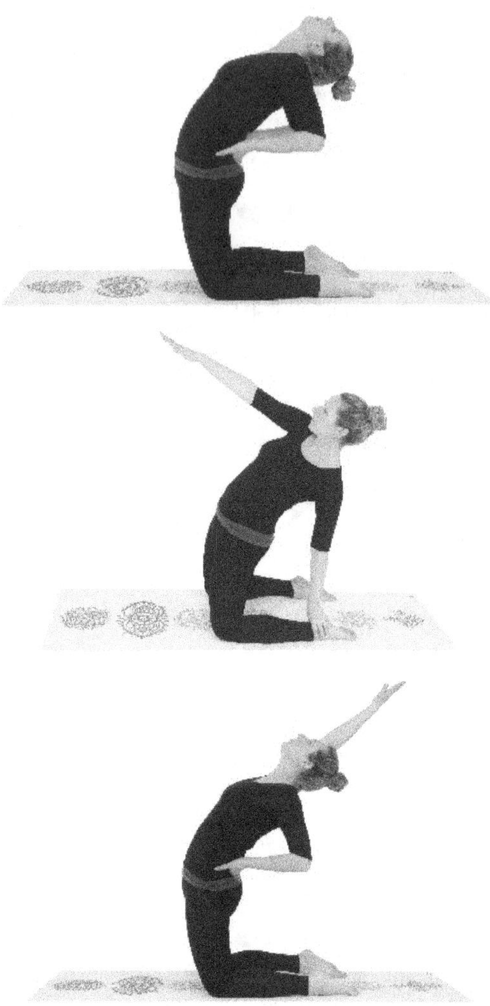

6. Inhale to come to table top position. Exhale, tuck your toes inside and adjust your body to Parvatasana.

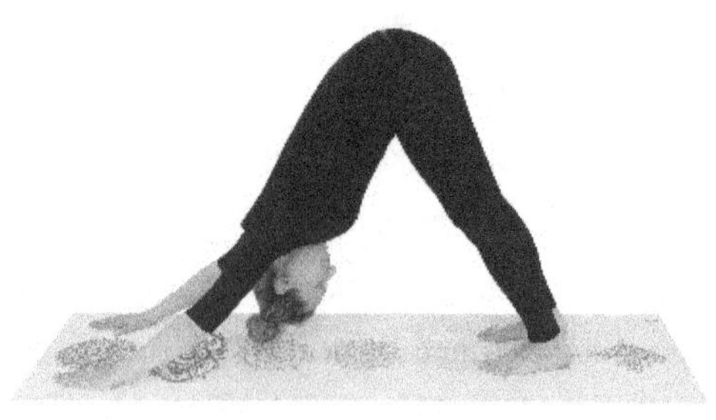

7. Inhale to Ardha Chandrasana.

8. Exhale while still looking forward to get into Ashwa Sanchalanasana.

9. Inhale, with the chest forward, fixing the gaze straight and place the hands on the shins into Ardha Uttanasana. If support is needed to go deeper to the ground, two yoga blocks can be used, one per hand to hold.

10. Exhale, bend from the hips to Vayu Nishkasana.

11. Inhale, bend your knees a bit and lift yourself up, let your hands reach forward and come to the modified.

12. Exhale, get back to Pranamasana and then place one hand on the heart and the other on the belly.

52. Equal Standing Pose – Samasthiti

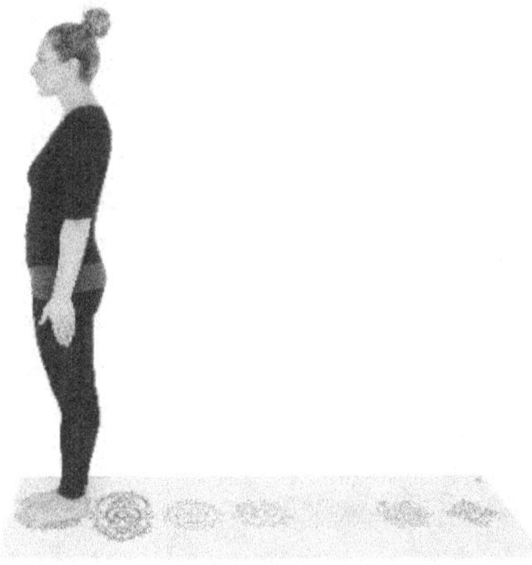

Practice: It is a basic standing pose with the feet together and the body upright. The hands are parallel to the sides of the body, with the palms facing or touching the sides of the glutes.

Breathing: Normal breathing.

Awareness: Physical – on breathing and whole body relaxation. Spiritual – on sacral (swadhisthana) chakra or root (mooladhara) chakra.

Benefits: Improves the body posture and relaxes the body muscles.

Precautions: Since it is a standing asana and may be required to stand for some time, those with recent surgery or conditions in the areas of knees, hips or spine should not practice.

53. Prayer Pose – Pranamasana

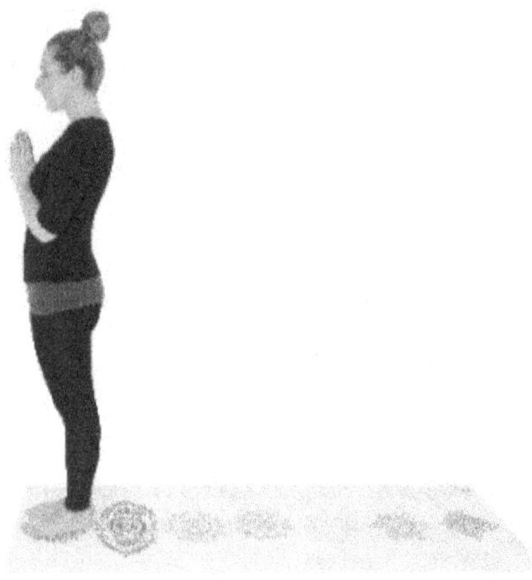

Practice: From Samasthiti, open the feet at hip-width or more than that for better balance, especially after second trimester. Bring the palms of the hands together in Namaste Mudra and breathe normally. This asana is performed in the beginning and in the end of Surya Namaskar practices; it can also be performed between asanas to find balance and concentrate before consuming practice.

Breathing: Normal breathing.

Awareness: Physical – on breathing and keeping the palms in front of the chest. Spiritual – on sacral (swadhisthana) chakra or root (mooladhara) chakra.

Benefits: Increases balance and concentration. Calms the mind and relieves from stress and anxiety.

54. Raised Arms Pose – Hasta Utthanasana

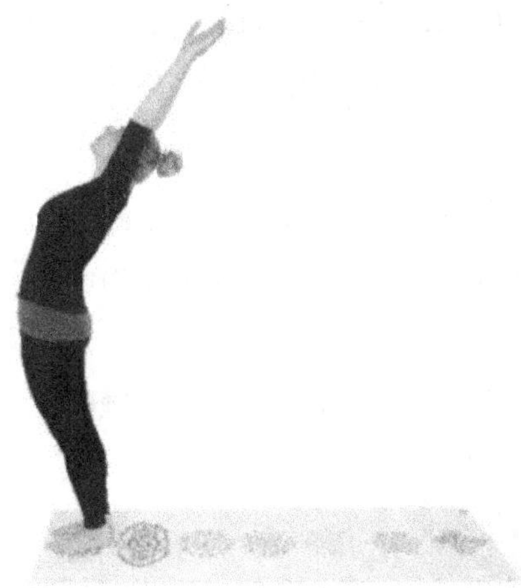

Practice: With the hands separated and raised above the head, stretch the arms upwards and backwards. Simultaneously, tilt the head and upper trunk slightly backwards.

Modification:

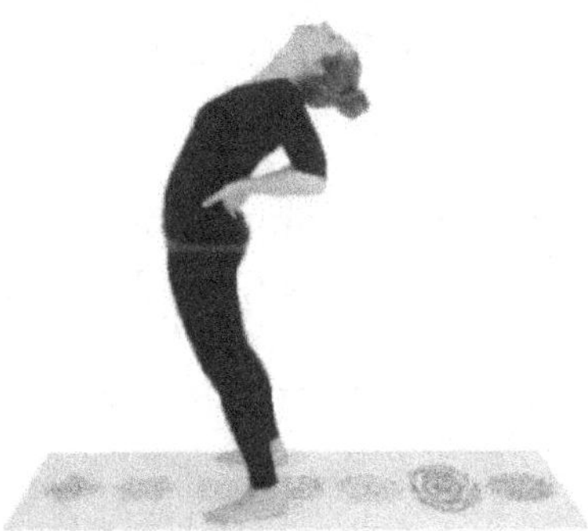

To avoid imbalance with the back bend or overstretching the abdomen especially from second trimester onwards, it is advisable to turn the palms inwards, bend the elbows and place the hands close to the sides of lower back to support the back.

Breathing: Inhale on raising the arms.

Awareness: Physical – on stretching the abdomen muscles and expanding the lungs. Spiritual – on throat (vishuddhi) chakra.

Benefits: Stretches the abdomen muscles. Stretches and tones the arms and shoulders. Strengthens the legs. Opens up the chest, expands the lungs and benefits the respiratory system. Helps to stretch the spine and strengthen the spinal extensors.

Precautions: Those with spinal, back, hip joints or ankles conditions, and sciatica or abdominal hernia should avoid the practice.

55. Hand to Foot Pose – Padahastasana

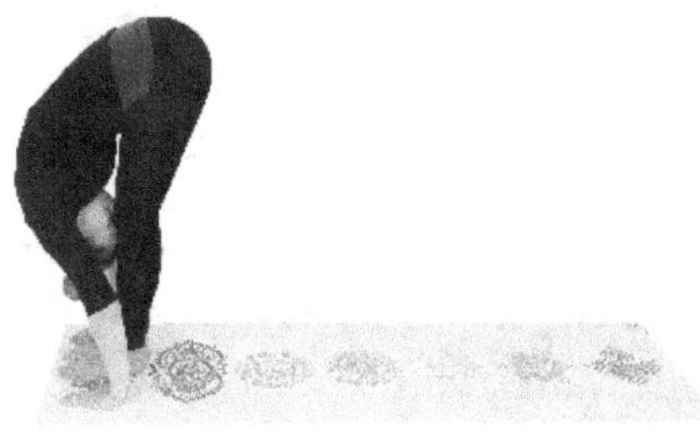

Practice: From Hasta Utthanasana bend forward from the hips for the fingers or the palms to touch the ground, by the side of each foot. The forehead should come as close to the knees as it feels comfortable, and the knees should be straight.

Breathing: Exhale on forward bending. Contract the abdomen when in final position to exhale as much air as possible from the lungs.

Awareness: Physical – on breathing and on the back and pelvis. Spiritual – on sacral (swadhisthana) chakra.

Benefits: Massages the digestive organs, therefore relieves from flatulence, constipation, or indigestion. Strengthens the spinal nerves. Can improve concentration and metabolism.

Precautions: Those with back conditions should only bend to maximum 90° degree angle only, or bend only to the point they feel comfortable; or can try instead Ardha Uttanasana instead.

Note: Can be practiced only until 10-12 gestational week and after fourth trimester given the physical body is fully recovered from childbirth. During a pregnancy, it is advisable to practice the final position of Vayu Nishkasana instead, which will put less pressure on the abdomen area.

56. Half Forward Bend – Ardha Uttanasana

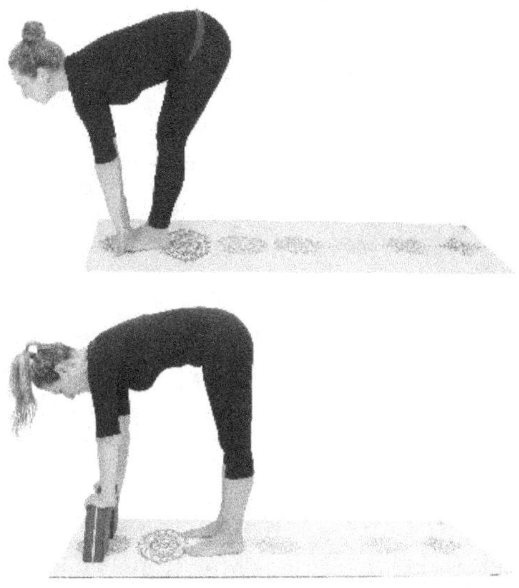

Practice: From Hasta Utthanasana, inhale to lengthen the torso and exhale to bend forward from the hips, keeping the spine straight, until the back forms a 90° degree angle with the legs. From second trimester onwards, can use the support of a yoga block per hand to avoid deeper bending and any belly compression.

Variation 1:

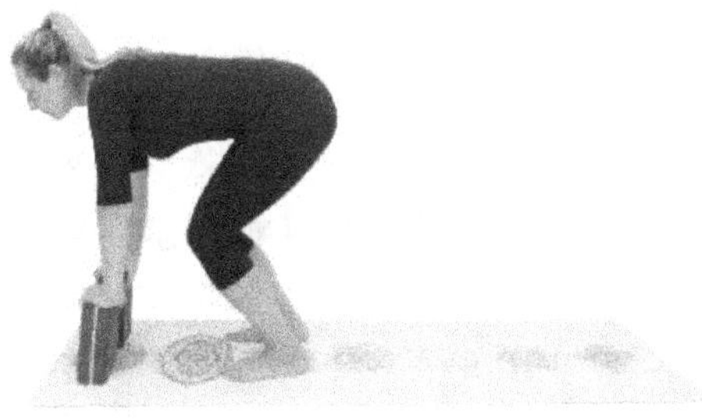

When at the final position, can perform gentle squats while holding the position with normal breathing.

Variation 2:

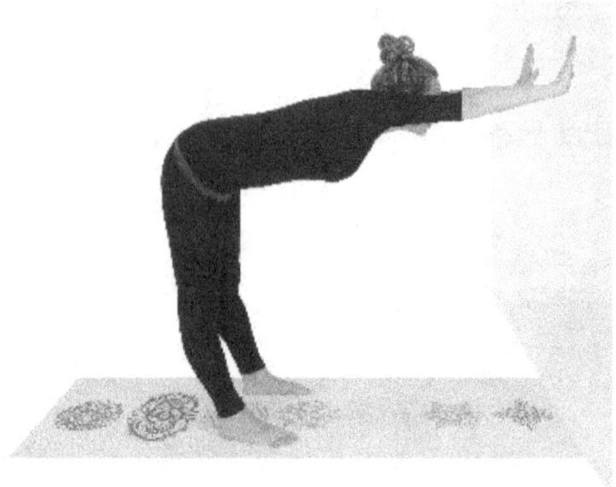

During the third trimester, previous variations may not be feeling comfortable due to the growing belly. Instead, can practice – with less effects though, by coming to as much as possible to 90° degrees angle to a wall leaning forward position where the palms of the hands or the elbows are nicely pushing the wall away. The legs should be positioned wide apart to comfort level and be straight. If legs are aligned with the hips, the stretch will be sensed to the forearms, shoulder blades and middle back. If legs are positioned slightly in front of the perineum with the tailbone pushed away from the body creating a gentle spinal curve, stretch will be sensed to the whole arm, shoulder blades and all the way to lower back.

Breathing: Inhale to lengthen the torso. Exhale to bend. Normal breathing at the position. Inhale to return to position.

Awareness: Physical – on breathing and on stretching the hamstrings, back and spinal cord. Spiritual – on sacral (swadhisthana) chakra.

Benefits: Massages the digestive organs, relieves from flatulence, constipation, or indigestion. Stretches and strengthens the vertebrae nerves, back and spine to improve body posture; hamstrings and calves' muscles; front and back torso. Can improve concentration and metabolism.

Precautions: Those with spinal, lower back or hamstrings conditions should avoid this practice.

57. Equestrian Pose – Ashwa Sanchalanasana

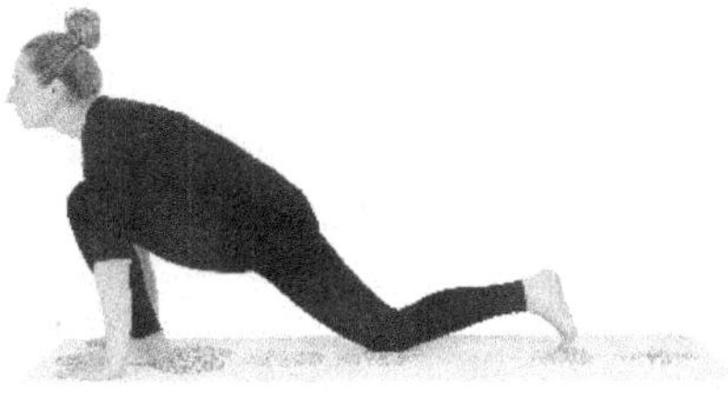

Practice: From Padahastasana or Ardha Uttanasana place the hands on the ground near the feet. Extend and stretch the right leg backward for as far as it feels comfortable or extend and keep the knee in contact with the ground, and grasp the floor with the toes. Simultaneously, bend the left knee with the sole of the foot flat on the ground diagonally open on the outer side of the left shoulder to avoid belly compression. The arms should be straight. The body weight should be supported by the hands, bent foot, extended knee and the toes of the extended leg. The head can look straight for those suffering from dizziness or nausea; or titled slightly backward gazing just above the eyebrow center with the back arched.

Variation: With the Baby

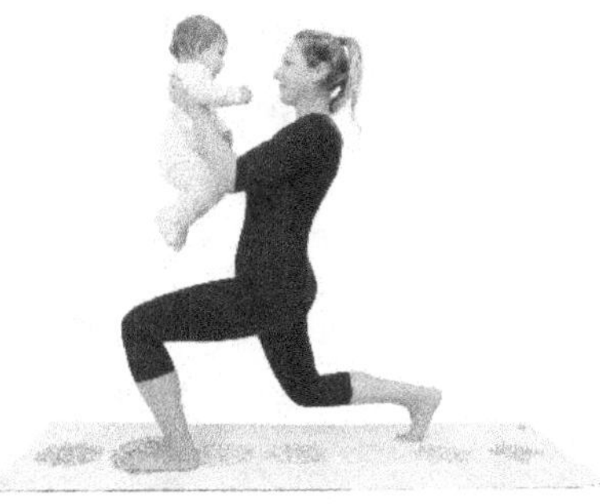

When co-practicing with the baby, similarly, can do a *High Lunge Pose – Utthita Ashwa Sanchalanasana,* which varies on the positioning of the arms being overhead normally. Hold firmly the baby in front of your chest by holding the positioning of the arms in front of the chest. The movement should be only on the back leg, which is bending from the knee to high or low lunges according to personal physique and holding the balance safely for both mum and baby.

Breathing: Inhale to stretch the leg back. Normal breathing when holding the position.

Awareness: Physical – on feeling the stretch from the thigh to the lower back, and at final balancing position place awareness on the eyebrow center.

Benefits: Stretches and strengthens the hip and psoas muscles, the quadriceps, gluteus maximus and hamstrings on the extended leg. Stretches the calf muscles of the front leg.

Precautions: Those with injuries in the areas of hips, knees, ankles, shoulders, wrists, neck or spinal column should avoid this asana. Should not attempt over-curving the spine to avoid overstretching the abdominal muscles. The extended leg should be extended as far as it feels comfortable, regardless if the knee is in contact with the ground. If there is a perineum or symphysis pubic pain this asana should not be practiced.

Note: Could be practiced only during a normal pregnancy by an experienced practitioner. From second trimester onwards, awareness should be put on not compressing the belly when coming into position, and have no jerky movement when coming out of the position. If practicing with the knee in contact with the ground, can use a folded blanket to reduce pressure on the knee joints. Post childbirth, practice only after the physical body has totally recovered.

58. Half Moon Pose – Ardha Chandrasana

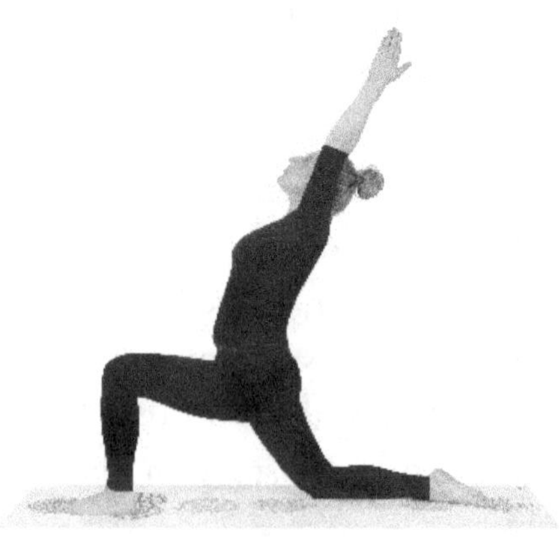

Practice: From Ashwa Sanchalanasana balance, and inhale to raise and stretch the arms above the head with the arms at shoulder width apart. Raise the chin slightly, tilt the head back, look up, and gently arch the back. If choosing to remain in that position, breathing should be normal. To come out from the position, exhale to lower the arms and return to Equestrian Pose.

Breathing: Inhale to raise the arms, tilt the head back and arching the back. Normal breathing while on position. Exhale to lower the arms.

Awareness: Physical – on normal breathing, balancing and controlling the movement. Spiritual – on throat (vishuddhi) chakra.

Benefits: Stretches the spinal cord and help on correcting body posture. Strengthens the spine, abdomen muscles and lower limb. Opens the chest area benefiting the respiratory system. Flexes the hamstrings and hips. Provides physical and mental balance and stability.

Precautions: Those suffering from low blood pressure or hernia, and having injuries in the areas of hips, knees, ankles, shoulders, wrists, neck or spinal column should avoid this asana. Should not attempt over-curving the spine to avoid overstretching the abdominal muscles. The lunge should be as wide as it feels comfortable. If there is a perineum or symphysis pubic pain this asana should not be practiced.

Note: Could be practiced at any phase of a normal pregnancy by an experienced practitioner with cautiousness.

59. Mountain Pose – Parvatasana

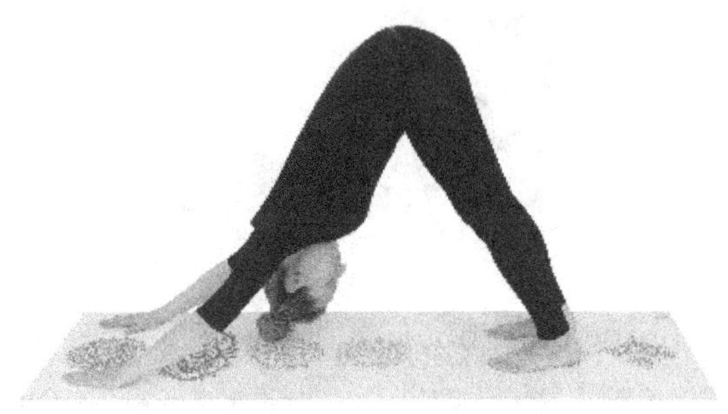

Practice: From Ashwa Sanchalanasana when practicing Surya Namaskar, or any other kneeling position, keep the hands under the shoulders, slowly extend one leg at a time, raise the buttocks, allow the head to follow the natural movement and be lowered between the forearms to come on an upside-down 'V' shape or mountain shape position. At the final position, normally target is to have arms and legs straight, heels touching the ground, the head and shoulder should be toward the knees. During a normal pregnancy, the movements and final position can be adjusted to width and extension that feels comfortable without putting much effort to touch the heels to the ground.

Breathing: Exhale to take each leg back. Normal breathing at the final position.

Awareness: Physical – on breathing and stretching from the Achilles' tendons (heels), to the back of lower limbs, shoulders and throat. Spiritual – on throat (vishuddhi) chakra.

Benefits: Strengthens and stretches the nerves and muscles in the legs, arms, shoulders and back. Helps circulation, particularly in the areas of upper spine and shoulder blades.

Precautions: Should be cautious with any inverted asanas during a pregnancy as these can have a reverse effect which can create acidity in the body, due to the baby weight pushing the stomach area.

60. Cobra Pose – Bhujangasana

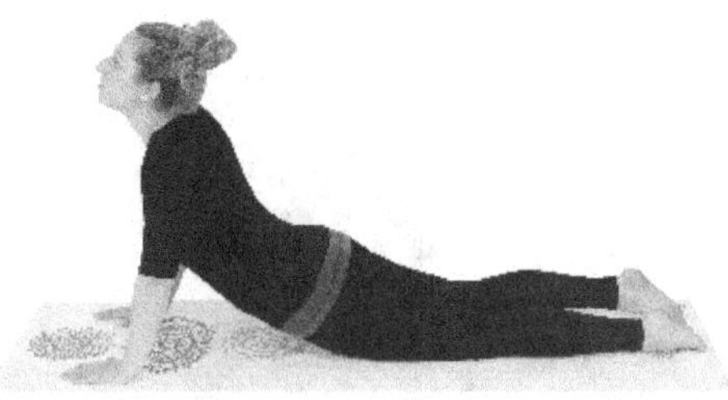

Practice: Lie on a prone position with the feet together or slightly apart to avoid strain in the lower back region. Place the palms on the sides of the breasts or shoulders and inhale to lift the upper body up. The hands should be stretched and the head slightly tilted backwards. The perineum should remain in contact with the ground. Remain at the position for 10-15 easy counts with normal breathing; or can hold the breath and engage the core on this position. Exhale to bend the hands by the elbows and lower the arms to return to starting position. This is 1 round. Can practice this 8-10 times during the classic Surya Namaskar.

Breathing: Inhale to raise the body. Normal breathing or holding the breath on the upward movement. Exhale to lower the body.

Awareness: Physical – on stretching the spine. Spiritual – on sacral (swadhisthana) chakra.

Benefits: Stretches the spine, chest, lungs, heart, shoulders and abdominal muscles. Tones the hip area. Relieves from lower back and sciatica pain.

Precautions: Those suffering from digestive disorders, hernia or hyperthyroidism should not practice this asana.

Note: No prone position asana should be practiced during pregnancy, especially after first trimester.

61. Striking Cobra Pose – Shashank Bhujangasana

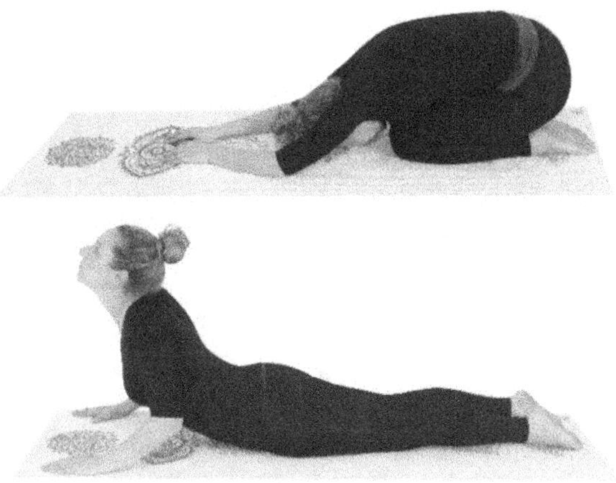

This pose is a combination of Child's Pose – Shashankasana and Cobra Pose – Bhujangasana. Start the flow with Child's Pose and slowly move to Bhujangasana. Repeat 5-10 times.

Breathing: Inhale on Bhujangasana. Exhale on Shashankasana.

Awareness: Sacral Chakra (Swadhisthana)

Benefits: Same as Shashankasana and Bhujangasana. The combination though is an excellent asana to tone the abdominal and pelvic region, which make it ideal for post-natal practicing.

Precautions: Same as Shashankasana and Bhujangasana.

Note: To be practiced after the fourth trimester.

Seated Asanas & Forward Bends

As explained previously, it is recommended to sit in Sukhasana while practicing any seated asanas during the prenatal period. From second trimester onwards the heel should not touch the belly and should create some space between the heel, perineum and belly to sit comfortably.

The following asanas can be considered as seated warm up or cooling down practices.

62. Head to Knee Pose – Janu Sirshasana

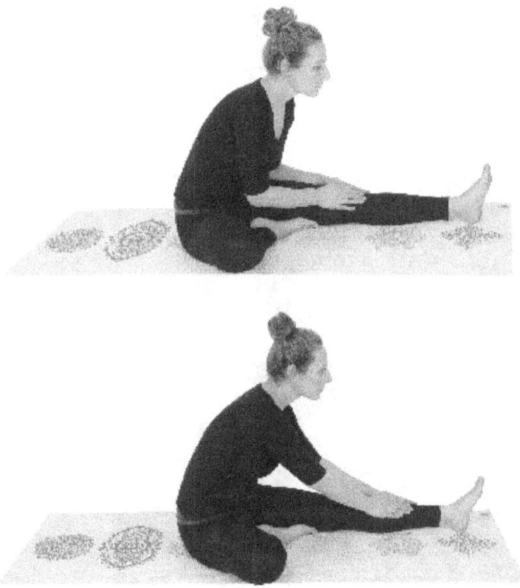

Practice: Very softly bend one knee and gently rest it on the floor while bringing the sole closer to the perineum and against the inner thigh. The spine should be straight throughout the whole practice. Inhale to bring hands up parallel to the ears. While exhaling, bend from the hip joint the upper body by bringing it to the level where hands are rested on the knee or shin bone. To return back to original position, slowly inhale to bring hands up and exhale to bring the hands down. Stay in the position for 3 normal breaths and return to the starting position. Can repeat 3-5 times with each leg.

First Trimester: The extended leg must be open in a straight position in front of the body.

Second Trimester: The extended leg must be diagonally open so the growing belly is nicely accommodated.

Third Trimester: The extended leg must be wider diagonally open so the growing belly is nicely accommodated and not touching the thigh at any point during the practice.

Modification 1: With the hands on the thighs, inhale normally, control the movement from the hip joint and while exhaling slide down the leg slowly until the point where the upper body is straight and the hands are stretched on the shin bone. Stay in the position for 3 normal breaths and exhale to slide back up the leg to the starting position. Can repeat 3-5 times with each leg.

Modification 2:

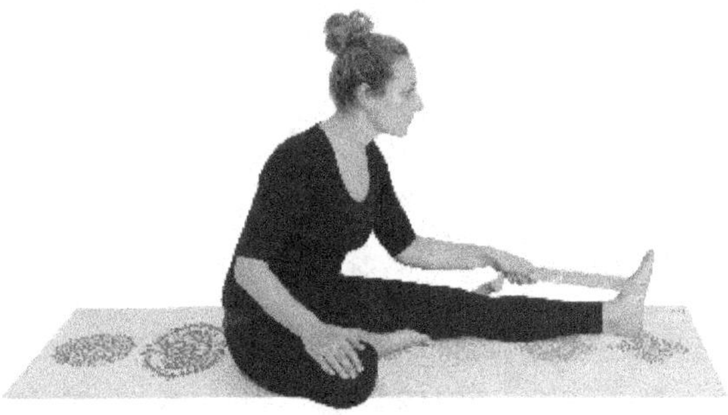

Can use a resistance thera-band or a long cloth by holding the two edges and fix the band at the arch of the extended foot. Sit up straight and slowly pull the band and walk towards the foot until the point the belly is not touching the thigh. Stay in the position for 3 normal breaths and return to the starting position.

Modification 3: With the baby

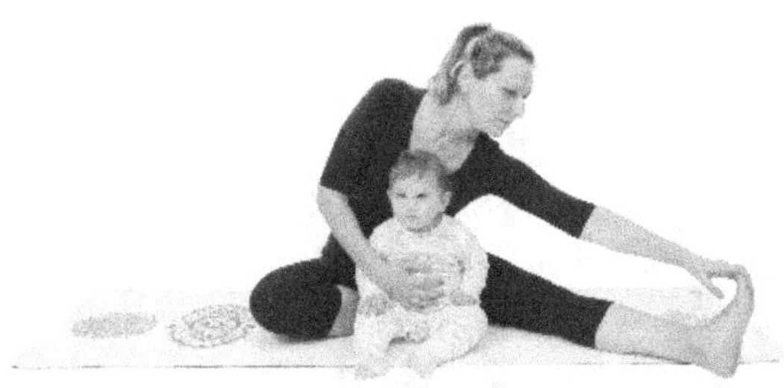

Co-practice this asana with the baby in the first year of motherhood. Practice will be more comfortable for both mother and baby with the extended leg diagonally open.

Breathing: Inhale to lift the hands up, exhale to bend and normal breathing at the final position when practicing during pregnancy. During the postnatal period, in the final position can hold breath for a comfortable length of time.

Awareness: In the physical level, intension is to stretch the back and leg region muscles with normal breathing on final position. In the spiritual level, swadhisthana (sacral) chakra is activated.

Benefits: Even by half bending to the knee or shin bone, stretches the back, the hamstring and cuff muscles. Stimulates circulation to the nerves and posterior muscles of the spinal cord. Loosens up the legs in preparation for meditation asanas.

Precautions: Should not be practiced by people with severe back conditions, sciatica or hernia.

Note: No jerky movement should occur in any part of the body, especially in the abdomen area. At any time, do not hold the breath. Only getting to the position is with breath awareness during pregnancy practicing. The intention is not to achieve flexibility, but build strength to the body. Practitioner should go until the point there is no strain, and not to achieve the final bend. The movement should not have a compression effect in any part of the abdomen area.

63. Spiraled Head to Knee Pose – Parivritti Janu Sirshasana

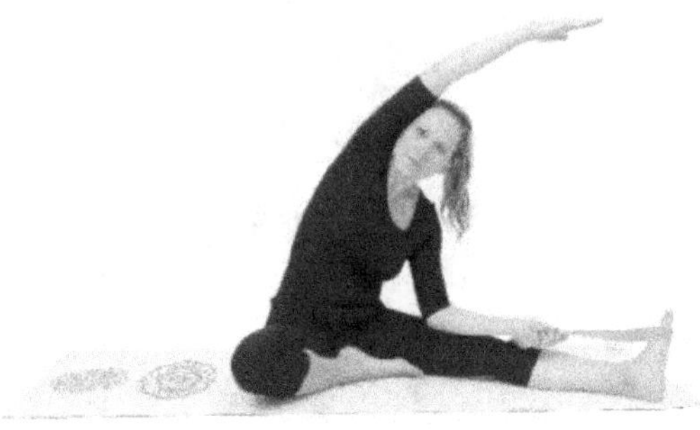

Practice: Starting pose same as Janu Sirshasana with the use of thera-band and the extended leg diagonally open. Maintain a good grip on the thera-band and rest the elbow on the thigh. Inhale to bring the hand up. Exhale to lateral bending to the side of the extended leg. The limit of the bending is until the point the belly is not compressed. Stay in the position for 3 normal breaths and return to the starting position, lower the raised hand. Can repeat 3-5 times with each leg.

Modification: With the baby

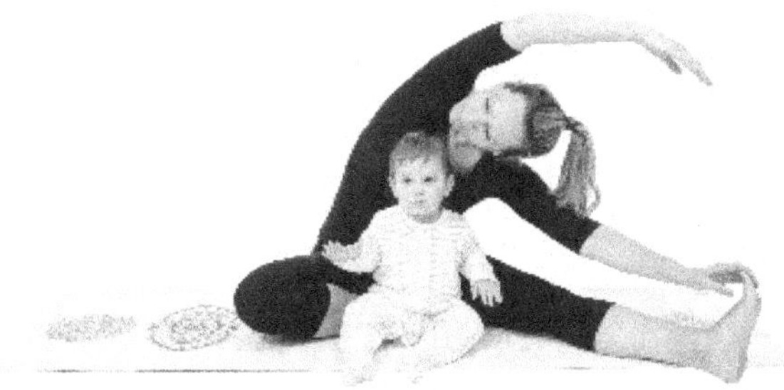

Can co-practice this asana with the baby in the first year of motherhood. Full bend may not be possible with baby sitting in front of the perineum. Though, can practice lateral bending.

Breathing: Inhale to lift the hand up, exhale to bend the body to the side and normal breathing at the final position when practicing during pregnancy. In the postnatal period, in the final position can hold breath for a comfortable length of time.

Awareness: Physical – on half lateral bending and body stretch. Spiritual – on solar plexus (manipura) chakra.

Benefits: Even by half bending, stretches the shoulder blades and the hamstring muscles. Loosens up the legs in preparation for meditation asanas.

Precautions: Should not be practiced by people with back conditions, sciatica or hernia. Only the modifications should be practiced during pregnancy.

Note: Would-be-mums should listen to their body and follow the instructions of the yoga teacher when practicing. No jerky movement should occur in any part of the body, especially in the abdomen area. At any time, do not hold the breath during pregnancy practicing. Only getting to the position is with breath awareness, on the final position there should be normal breathing. The intention is not to achieve flexibility, but build strength to the body. Practitioner should go until the point there is no strain, and not to achieve the final bend. The movement should not have a compression effect in any part of the abdomen area.

64. Back Stretching Pose – Paschimottanasana

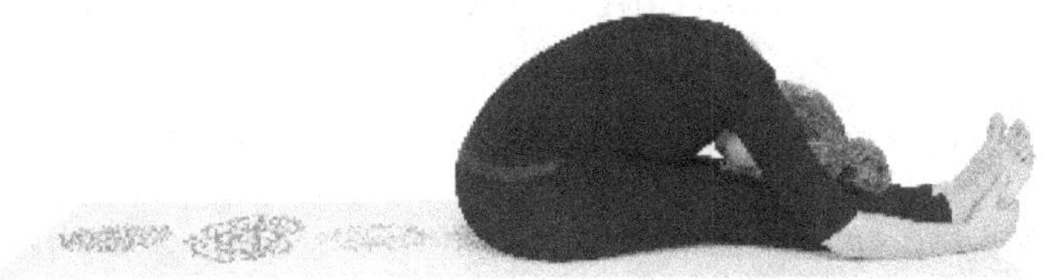

Practice: Sit with the legs outstretched, feet together and bring the hands on the knees. Normal breathing to relax the body, and slowly bend forward from the hips and slide down the hands to the legs. Try to touch the toes with the hands, and the knees with the nose or forehead. Do not strain; position must feel comfortable. Gently return to the starting position. This is 1 round and can practice up to 5 rounds if practitioner is a beginner, or up to 5 minutes for advanced practitioners.

Modification:

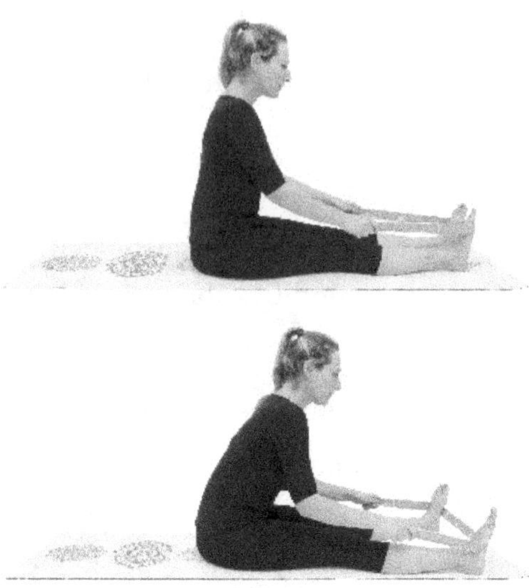

Breathing: Inhale in starting position. Exhale to bend. Normal breathing if holing position for larger duration, or hold the breath if staying on position for small duration. Inhale to return to starting position.

Awareness: Physical – on breathing and on the core area, stretching the back and leg muscles. Spiritual – on pelvic (swadhisthana) chakra.

Benefits: Stretches the hamstrings and flexes the hip joints. The whole abdominal and pelvic region organs get strengthened and massaged. Stimulates blood flow to the spinal nerves and muscles.

Precautions: Not to be practiced by those who suffer from severe back conditions, sciatica or hernia.

Note: Can be practiced only after the body has recovered from childbirth, maybe towards the end of fourth trimester onwards, and depending if baby was born by caesarian section. In that case, aim is still not to compress the abdomen area, at least, not until stiches are dropped and wound has completely healed. If practitioner is unable to touch the toes, can use a thera-band or a rope to hold onto. As a warm-up for this asana, can practice Janu Sirshasana and Janu Naman.

65. Wide Angled Seated Forward Bend – Upavistha Konasana

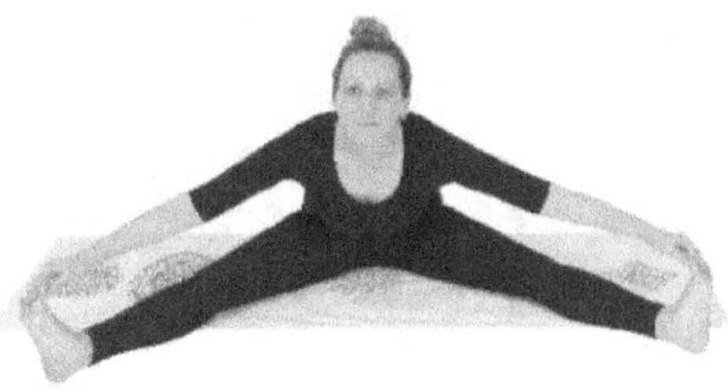

Practice: Sit with the legs spread apart as wide as possible with the spine erect. Exhale to lean forward the trunk to touch the toes with the hands. Continue normal breathing without any compression on the belly. Inhale to return to upright position.

Modification:

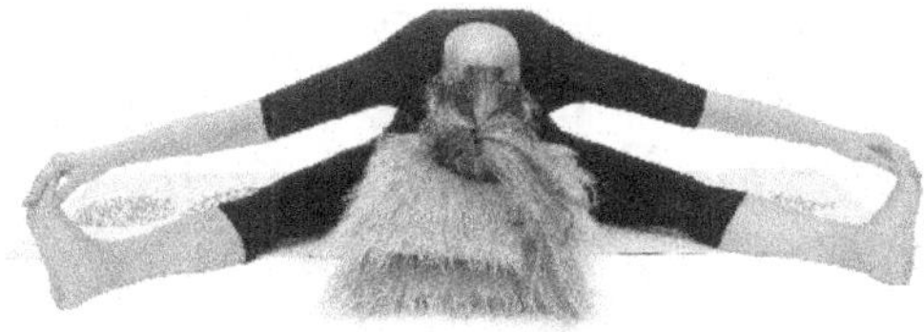

Have 2 or 3 cushions one on top of the other in front of the body. For advanced practitioners on their second trimester onwards with no pregnancy complications, full bend can be done, with the forehead resting on the cushions while touching the toes, as long as there is no belly compression. Without holding the breath, stay in that position for 2 or 3 normal breaths, inhale to come up to upright position and release the arms.

Variation:

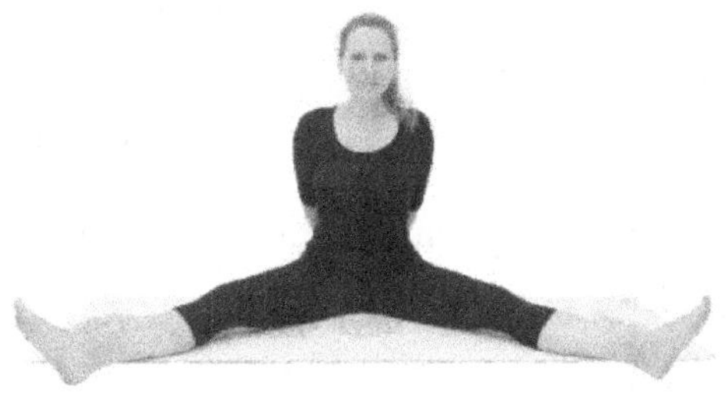

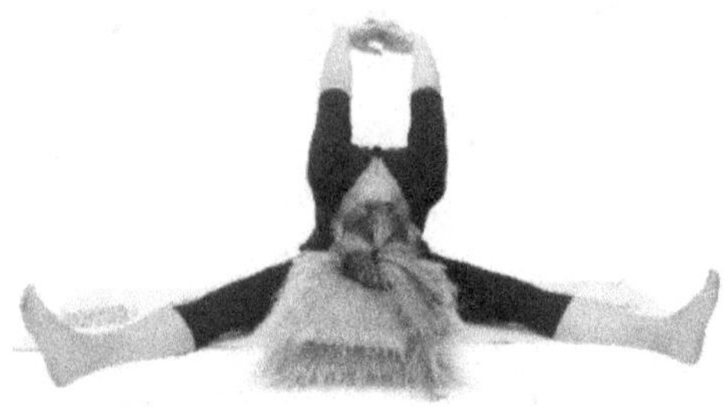

Sit with the legs spread apart as wide as possible with the spine erect. Interlock the fingers behind the back, and lean forward until the point the breath is comfortably normal. Half forward bend is recommended through pregnancy. Hands should remain close to the buttocks. For advanced practitioners with no pregnancy complications, full bend can be done, with the forehead resting on 2-3 cushions while raising the arms behind the back with no strain. Without holding the breath, stay in that position for 2 or 3 breaths, inhale to come up to upright position and lower the arms. If you like, in this modified pose, to lean forward, place the palms of the hands close to the inner thighs for a nice spinal stretch and maintain the balance.

Variation: With the Baby

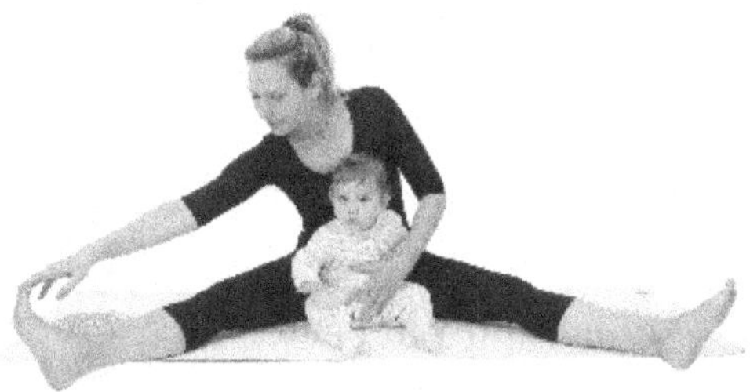

With your feet widely open, hold the baby with one hand and extend the other arm in an attempt to touch your toes. The forward bend should be from the hips and both buttocks should remain in touch with the ground.

Breathing: Inhale in starting position. Exhale to bend forward. Inhale to return to starting position.

Awareness: Physical – on the stretch of the legs, back, spine, shoulders and arms with continuous breathing. Spiritual – on root (mooladhara) chakra or sacral (swadhisthana) chakra.

Benefits: Stretches the hamstrings and increase flexibility in the hip joints. Encourages circulation to the nerves and muscles of the spine.

Precautions: Those with hernia or back conditions should not practice this asana.

Note: It is recommended to be practiced from second trimester onwards. On third trimester, may use a soft cushion between the belly and the ground to support the belly. While leaning forward, maintain the length of the spine. Forward bend should be until the point the breath is comfortably normal and there is no belly compression.

66. Seated Twist or Marichi Pose – Marichyasana

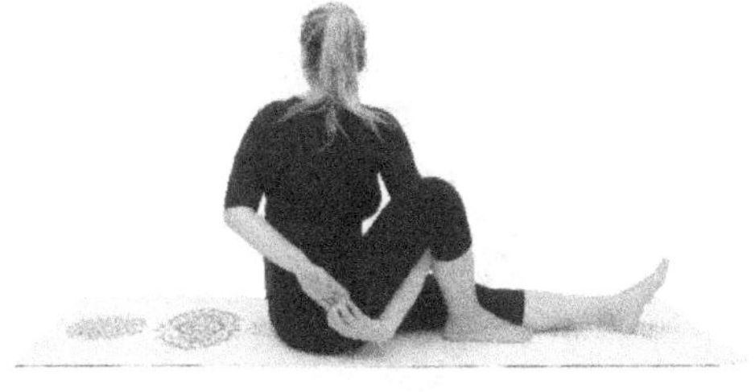

Practice: Starting from Base Position, bend the right knee and bring it closer to the body, a little higher than the knee level of the extended leg. Inhale to raise the right hand up, and while exhaling rotate the hand down and around the right knee or inside and between the hamstring and the back of the knee. Bring the left hand around the back aiming to touch the right hand, and then look back to the left shoulder to experience a mild twist on the spine and back. Breathe normally in the final position for 10 easy and fast counts. Inhale to release the pose slowly. Repeat the same with the other side. This is 1 round and can practice 3-5 rounds with normal breathing on the final position.

Modification 1:

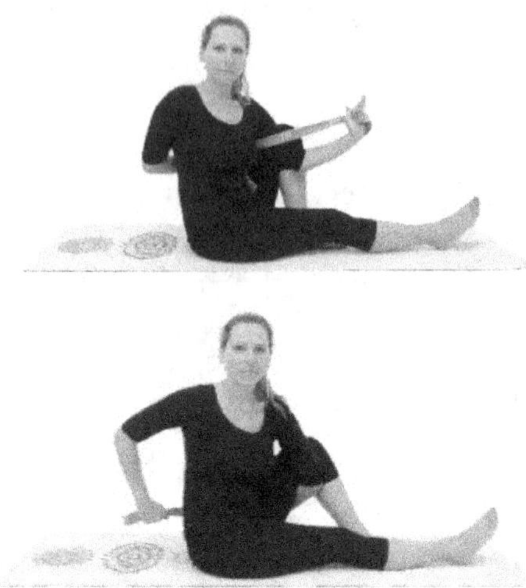

If not comfortable to touch hands, can use a cloth, cord or a thera-band for support.

Modification 2:

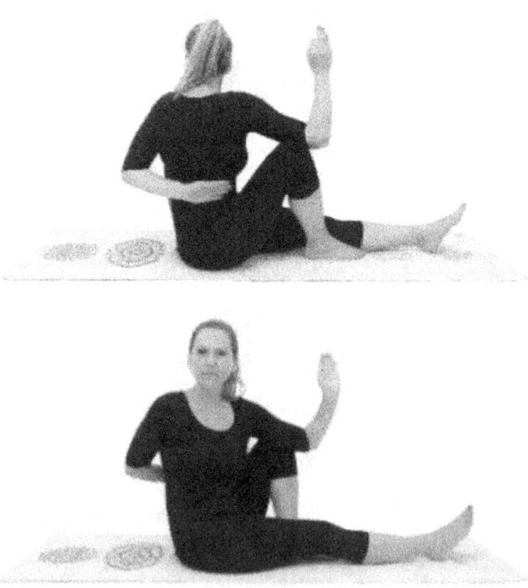

If no cloth, cord or thera-band is available, that is fine, the aim of the asana is to have the chest open twist and not the holding hands. In that case, place the right elbow on the bent right knee cap and bring the left hand from behind to rest on the right side obliques. Repeat the same with the other side.

Modification 3:

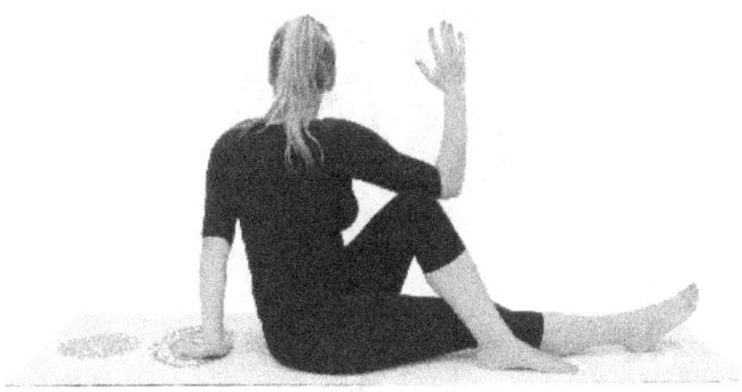

If Modification 2 is still challenging, ask practitioner to place left palm of the hand on the ground, to the side and slighly back of the buttocks, and perform soft opening twists per side.

Breathing: Normal breathing in the final position.

Awareness: Physical – on breathing and twisting only as far as it is comfortable, avoiding any compression of the belly. Spiritual – on solar plexus (manipura) chakra or sacral (swadhisthana) chakra.

Benefits: This asana is very good to be practiced during the whole pregnancy and fourth trimester because it stretches the back, elevates tension and stiffness around the vertebral column. Works as a chest opener.

Precautions: During pregnancy, and especially from late second trimester onwards, twist must be gentle and open with no belly compression. Positioning of the legs must be wider open to accommodate move. Those with back injury, rotator cuff should avoid practice, as well as those with weak wrists or injuries if holding position like Modification 3.

Note: In Ashtanga Yoga we can find many variations for Marichyasana, herein only the safest ones are given for pre and postnatal practicing.

67. Seated Prayer Flow – Sukhasana Namaste Hands Vinyasa

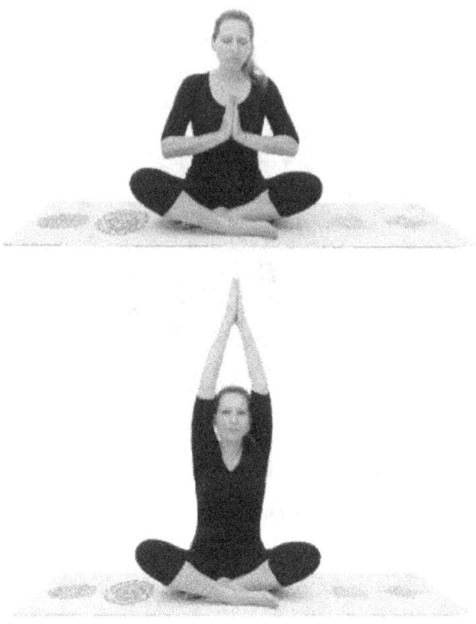

Practice: Sit in Sukhasana with the hands in Namaste Mudra in front of the chest. With spine erect and head straight, close the eyes, connect with the breath, connect with the body, connect with the mind. When ready, open the eyes and on inhalation open the hands smoothly to the sideways of the body to bring the hands upwards and above the head, connect the palms in anjali mudra and on exhalation, bring the hands down in front of the chest. Continue practicing for 8-10 rounds.

Breathing: Inhale to raise the arms. Exhale to lower the arms. Continuous breathing with the movement.

Awareness: Physical – synchronization of breath and movement. Spiritual – on heart (anahata) chakra.

Benefits: Stretches the chest, shoulder blades, upper back and triceps. Can help frozen shoulders relief.

Precautions: Those with injuries on the shoulders, back or spine should avoid practicing the vinyasa.

68. Seated Palm Tree Pose – Parvatasana in Sukhasana

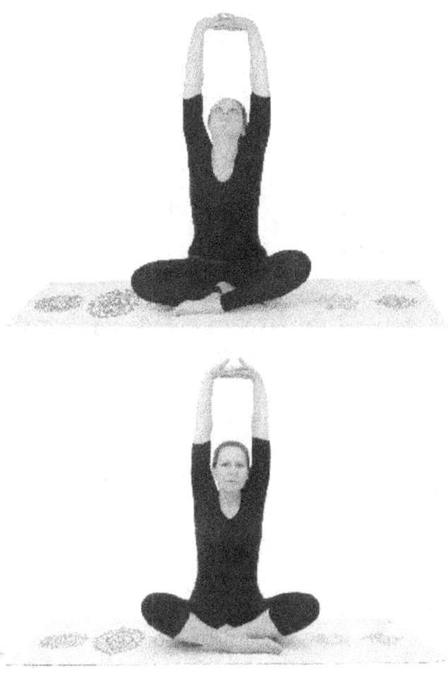

Practice: Sit in Sukhasana with the spine erect. Interlock the fingers and inhale to lift arms above the head with palms facing the ceiling. Fix the gaze either looking at the fingers above the head or straight. This is the starting position. Stay in the position for 5-10 normal breaths. Can repeat 2 sets of the same.

Variation:

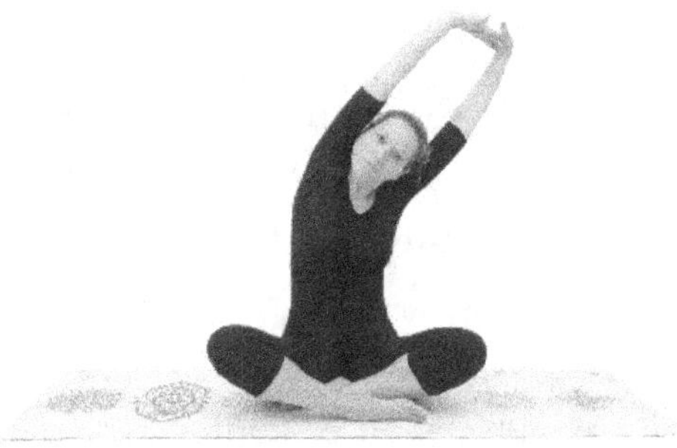

From starting position, exhale to bend sideways towards the left to feel the stretch on the side of the right rib cage. Inhale to return to the center.

Exhale to bend sideways to the right. Inhale to return to the center. This is 1 round and can practice 3-6 rounds.

Breathing: Inhale to raise the hands. Exhale to bend. Inhale to the center.

Awareness: Physical – on body alignment and synchronization of breath with the movement. Spiritual – on heart (anahata) chakra, solar plexus (manipura) chakra or sacral (swadhisthana) chakra.

Benefits: This is the lateral bending for the intercostal muscles. Can also benefit the muscles in arms and shoulders, chest, back and vertebrae, knees, psoas. Can release tension in the neck, help balance the thyroid glands

Precautions: Those with sciatica, or severe conditions in the areas of neck, shoulders, back or knees should avoid this practice.

Note: Can gaze up to the hands when bending, however, if practitioner suffers from dizziness and nausea, it is advisable to look straight.

69. Seated Side Bend – Parsva Sukhasana

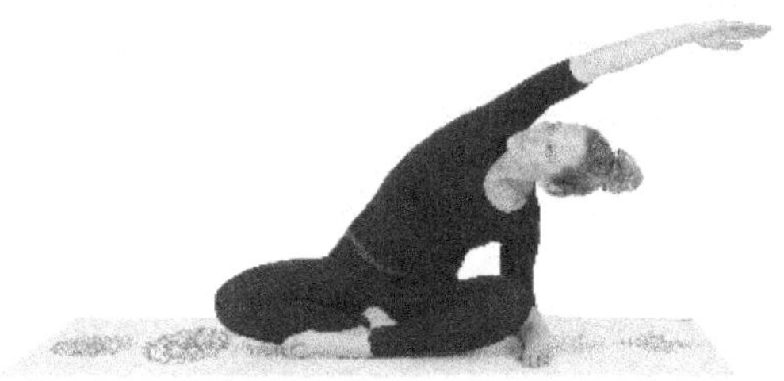

Practice: Sit in Sukhasana with both hands at the knees. Position the left hand next to the body, slightly away from the left buttock, or have the lower limb flat on the ground next to the knee for maximum stretch during the pre-conception and fourth trimester. Inhale to raise the right arm up, bending the left elbow close to the rib cage and on exhalation bend sideways towards the left side. Hand can either be lengthened in a straight line or curved in. Inhale to come back to the center. Repeat the same with the other side to complete 1 round. Can practice 3-6 rounds.

Modification:

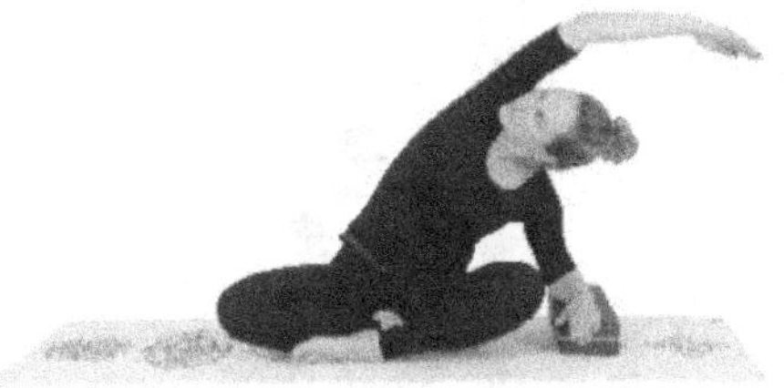

Those who find it difficult to have the lower limb flat on the ground, can use the support of a yoga block to lift up the body positioning.

Variation 1:

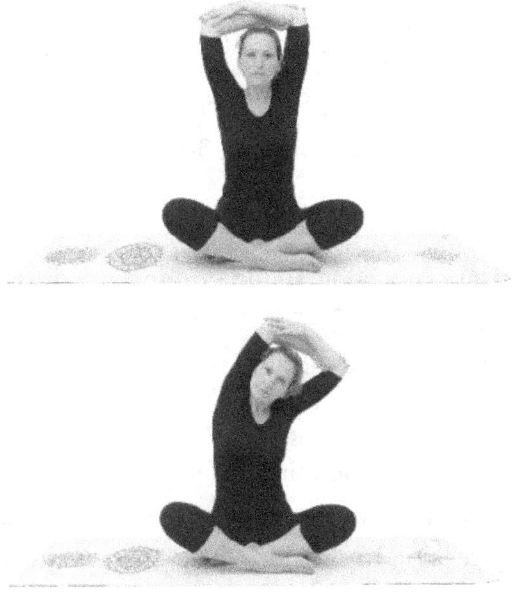

Inhale to take the hands up, exhale to bend the elbows and hold with each hand the opposite elbow. While breathing normally, feel the stretch in the chest region, fix the head between the inner upper arms. Exhale to bend sideways towards the left, inhale to the center, exhale to bend sideways towards the right, inhale to the center. This is 1 round and can practice 3-6 rounds.

Variation 2:

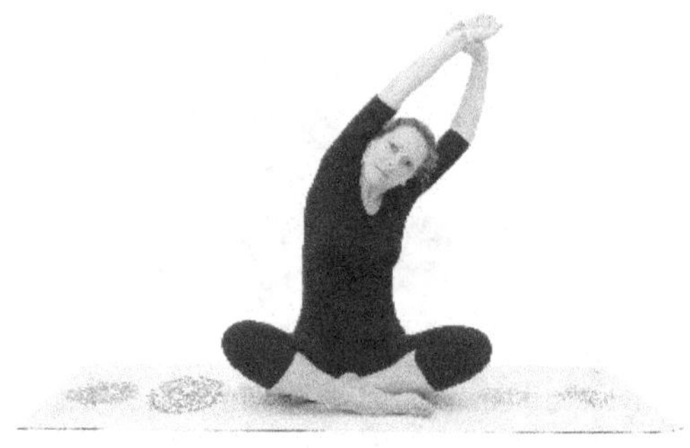

Inhale to raise both hands up with palms facing forward. With the left hand hold the wrist of the right hand to lengthen the arm. Exhale to bend sideways towards the left to feel the stretch on the side of the rib cage. Inhale to return to the center. Change hands – hold the left wrist with the right hand. Exhale to bend sideways to the right. Inhale to return to the center. This is 1 round and can practice 3-6 rounds.

Breathing: Inhale to raise the hands. Exhale to bend. Inhale to the center.

Awareness: Physical – on body alignment and synchronization of breath with the movement. Spiritual – on heart (anahata) chakra, solar plexus (manipura) chakra or sacral (swadhisthana) chakra and gentle activation of throat (vishuddhi) chakra.

Benefits: This is the lateral bending for the intercostal muscles. Can also benefit the muscles in arms and shoulders, chest, back and vertebrae, knees, psoas. Can release tension in the neck, help balance the thyroid glands

Precautions: Those with sciatica, or severe conditions in the areas of neck, shoulders, back or knees should avoid this practice.

Note: Practitioners during their pregnancy, and especially from second trimester onwards do not need to overstretch. A nice stretch can be achieved on the upper rib cage area even with a half bend. It is recommended to practice easy, rather than aiming to overstretch to reach the final position. The aim is not to touch the floor but feel the stretch to whichever level the body can feel.

70. Seated Spinal Twist – Parivritti in Sukhasana

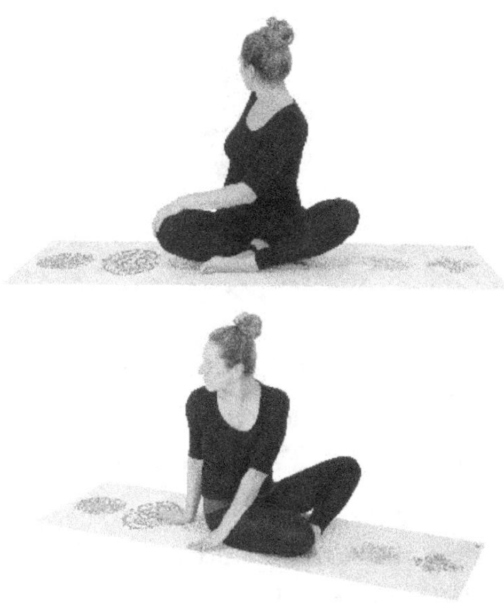

Practice: Sit in Sukhasana and inhale. Exhale to rest the right hand on the left knee. Inhale to round the left hand to the lower back or slightly away from the buttocks. The head should be turned towards the left shoulder. Exhale to return to the center. Repeat the same with the other side to complete 1 round. Can practice 3-6 rounds.

Breathing: Controlled breathing with the movement.

Awareness: Physical – on breath and stretching the chest, rib cage, upper back and shoulders. Spiritual – on sacral (swadhisthana) chakra) and root (mooladhara) chakra.

Benefits: This open twist stretches the hips, knees, ankles. Increases flexibility throughout the chest, shoulders and spinal cord and loosens the vertebrae. Releases tension on the posterior muscles. Helps to remove stress. Stimulates the diaphragm and digestive system. Can release mild backache which starts occurring from second trimester.

Precautions: Those with neck, shoulders, spine, lower back, hips, knees or pelvic floor conditions should only practice in the presence of an experienced yoga teacher.

71. Seated Eagle Pose – Garudasana

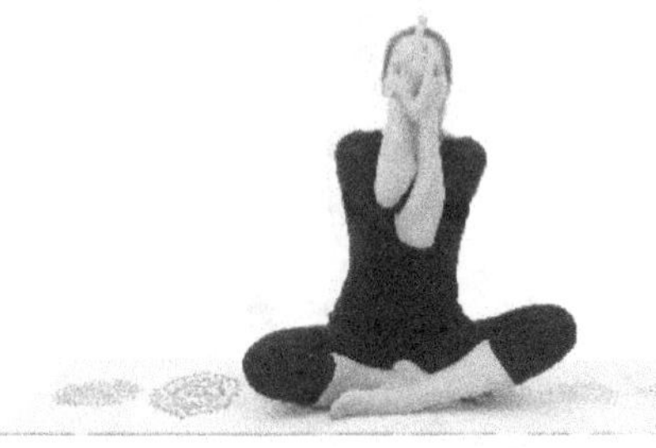

Practice: Inhale to bring the hands in front of the body and slowly round them with left elbow remaining below the right. Take the hands up slightly above the head and stay in that position comfortably for a few breaths and then slowly bring the hands down and release them. Change the hands so the right elbow is below the left one and repeat the same to complete 1 round. Can practice 3-6 rounds with normal breathing.

Breathing: Normal breathing.

Awareness: Physical – on stretching the shoulder blades. Spiritual on root (mooladhara) chakra or third eye (ajna) chakra.

Benefits: Stretches the shoulder blades as these are pulled away from each other with the rounded hands.

Precautions: Those with injuries on the wrists, elbows, shoulders or neck should avoid the practice.

Note: Garudasana is practiced with the legs and hands both rounded in the standing position, as a part of balancing asanas. During pregnancy, we separate the two rounded practices and we perform only the rounded hands while seated in Sukhasana. On standing position, we practice only the rounded legs. Especially from second trimester onwards when the breasts are getting larger, the rounded hands in front of the chest area may compress the breasts and give a feeling of tightness. In that case, the trunk should lean slightly forward to help the rounded hands be away from the breasts and belly. Practice can also be done seated in a chair with both soles on the ground.

72. Seated Cat & Cow Pose – Marjariasana

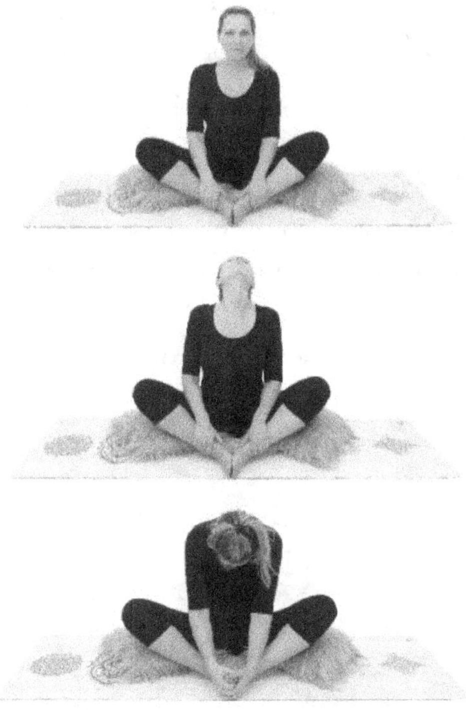

Practice: Sit in Full Butterfly – Poorna Titali Asana with the feet approximately 30cm or 1 foot away from the perineum. Use a cushion under each thigh or knee. The hands can be either on the ankles or on the toes. The back is erect. On inhalation, open the chest and look up with a mild curve on the back. On exhalation, drop the chin to the chest, and push the back gently away by rounding the back. This is 1 round. Can practice 3-6 rounds.

Variation 1:

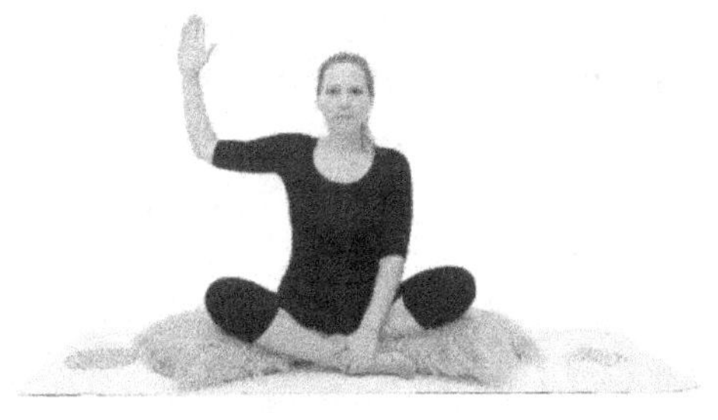

Sit in Sukhasana with supported thighs or knees by the use of cushions. Rest the hands on the floor in front of the body. Spine is in neutral erect position. On inhalation, open the chest and look up with a mild curve on the back. On exhalation, drop the chin to the chest, and push the back gently away by rounding the back. On next inhalation, when lifting the head up, lift the right hand also bent from the elbow to create a gentle curve in the back and feel the stretch on the chest, shoulder and entire upper arm area. On exhalation, bring the hand down and look down. Inhale to lift the head up and also lift the left hand. Exhale to bring the hand down and look down. This is 1 round. Can practice 3-6 rounds.

Variation 2:

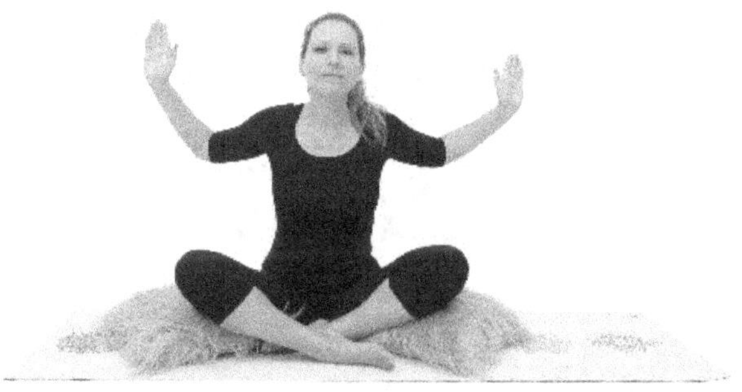

Sit in Sukhasana with supported thighs or knees by the use of cushions. Rest the hands on the ground in front of the body. Spine is in neutral erect position. On inhalation, open the chest and look up with a mild curve on the back. On exhalation, drop the chin to the chest, and push the back gently away by rounding the back. On next inhalation, when lifting the head up, lift to Cactus arms and exhale. Inhale to expand the chest, create a small curve in the back and feel the stretch on the chest, shoulder and entire upper arm area. Can be on that position for 10-15 easy counts with normal breathing. Inhale to exhale and bring the hands down on the ground in front of the body, look down with chin to the chest to a slight back bend. This is 1 round. Can practice 3-6 rounds.

Breathing: Synchronized breathing with the movement. Inhale to open the chest. Exhale to round the back.

Awareness: Physical – on stretching the chest, shoulder and entire upper arm area. Spiritual – on heart (anahata) chakra.

Benefits: Stretches the chest, shoulder and entire upper arm area. Depending on the seated position, the same benefits apply.

Precautions: Practitioners suffering from sciatica or pelvic conditions should only practice seated.

73. Seated Camel Pose – Ushtrasana in Sukhasana

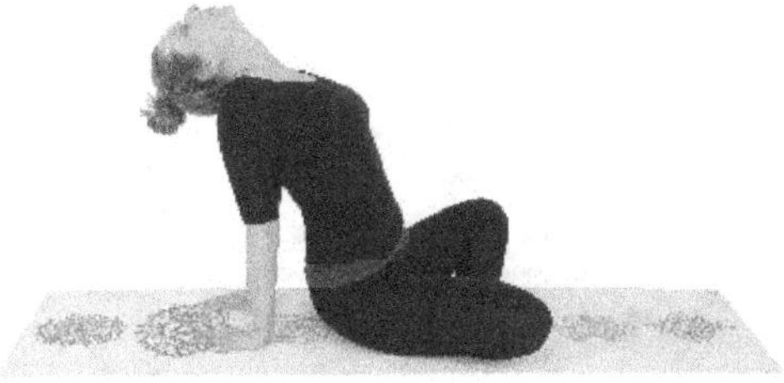

Practice: Sit in Sukhasana with the support of cushions under the knees if needed. Rest the hands on the ground behind the buttocks at a distance of practitioners' comfort. Spine is in neutral erect position. Inhale to move hands slightly further away from the buttocks and exhale. Inhale to expand the chest and create a gentle backward bend. Stay in that position with normal breathing for 10-15 easy counts. Inhale to exhale and bring the hands closer to the buttocks and gently bring the upper body back to the center. This is 1 round. Can practice 3-6 rounds.

Breathing: Normal breathing between the moves. Inhale to adjust hands behind the buttocks. Inhale to expand the chest. Exhale to come back to the center.

Awareness: Physical – on breathing and stretching the chest, shoulder blades, spinal cord and entire upper arm area. Spiritual – on heart (anahata) chakra.

Benefits: Stretches the chest, shoulder blades, spinal cord and entire upper arm area. Depending on the seated position, the same benefits apply.

Precautions: Not to be practiced by those with wrists conditions. Practitioners suffering from sciatica or pelvic conditions should only practice Ushtrasana seated.

74. Side-Reclining Leg Lift Pose – Anantasana

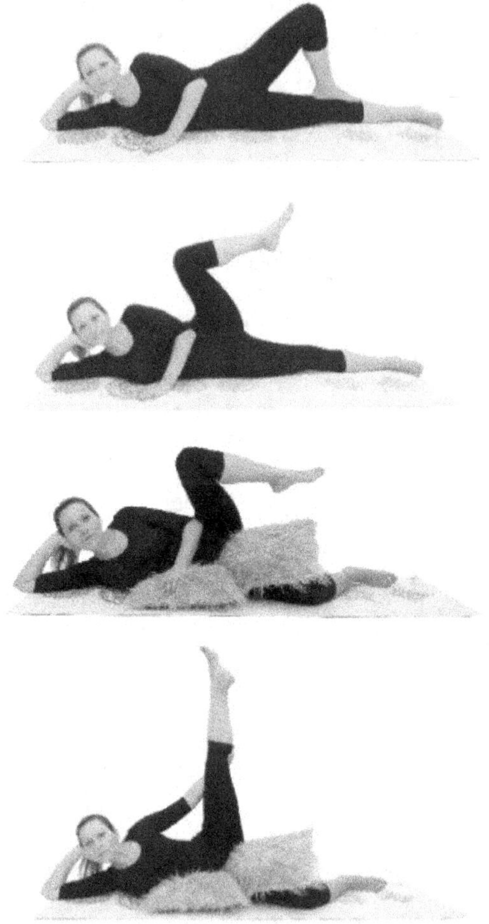

Practice: Similar position to Matsya Kridasana, lie on the right side and position the body comfortably with the legs either straight; or bent by the knees. Support the head with the palm of the right hand; or extend the right arm and rest the head on forearm. Use a cushion between the thighs and another between the belly and the ground from second trimester onwards. Find your body balance on the side by placing the left hand on the mat or on top of the cushion supporting the belly; can also place the soles against a wall for better stability. When balance is there, inhale to bend and open the leg wide to the side to a table-top position and slowly raise it up to 90°. To help the movement, can place the left hand on the cuff or hamstring on the upward movement. Exhale to slowly lower the leg back to table-top position and then to original position. Repeat the same for 8-12 counts and change sides.

Variation 1:

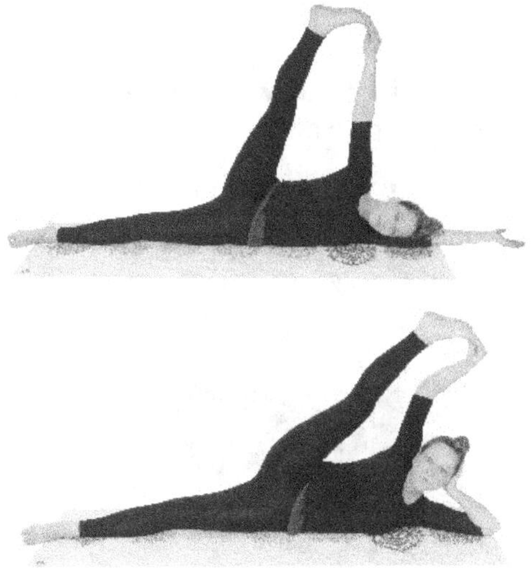

Starting with the knee bent at table top position, raise the leg by holding the toes where leg and arm should be extended. Repeat the same for 8-12 counts and change sides. When resting the head on the palm of the hand, the body gets inclined and the leg-lift can come closer to the body.

Modification:

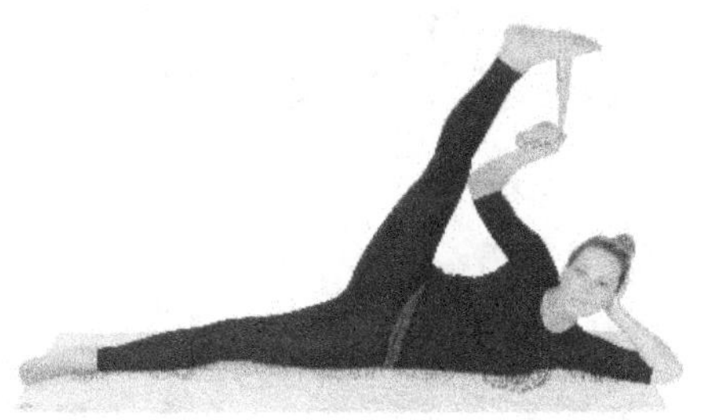

Can use the support of a thera-band if cannot reach to touch the toes with the fingers.

Variation 2:

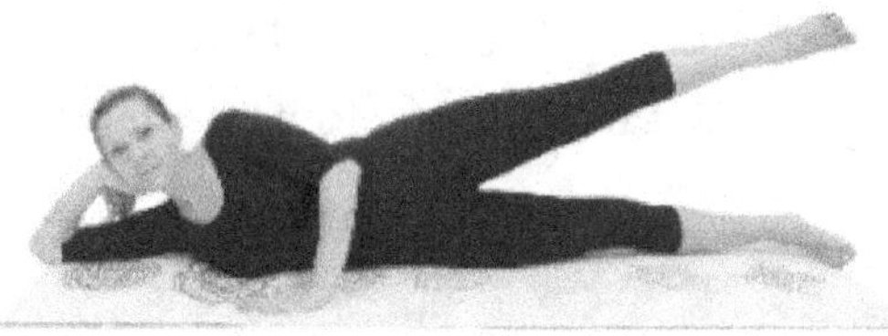

With the legs outstretched, either rest the head on the arm being extended beyond the head or hold the head with the palm of the hand. Place the other hand in front of the belly. Inhale to lift the leg up to 30° or 45° angle. Exhale to lower the leg. This is 1 round. Repeat the same for 8-12 counts and change sides.

Variation 3:

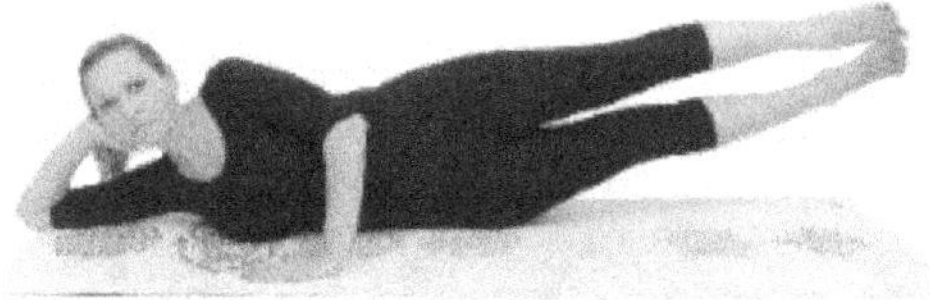

Similar to Variation 2, outstretch and lift the legs together while inhaling. On exhalation, lower the legs 10cm from the ground. This is 1 round. Repeat the same for 8-12 counts and change sides.

Variation 4:

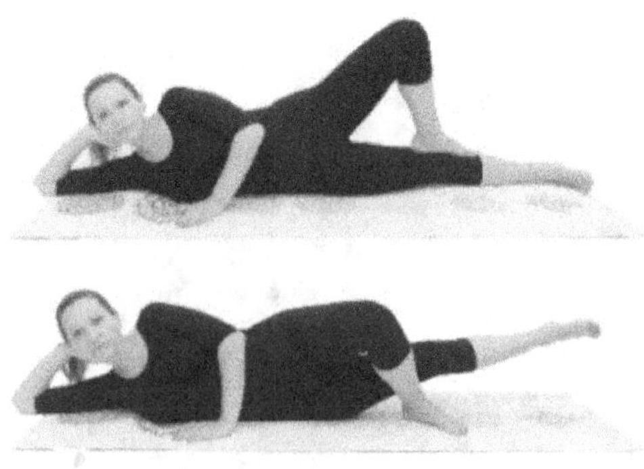

With the legs outstretched together on the ground, inhale to bend the top leg and rest it on cuff of grounded leg. Exhale to find the balance and adjust hands positioning with normal breathing. Inhale to cross over the top leg in front of the grounded knee or below the knee to avoid belly compression. Exhale and adjust body to balance with normal breathing. Inhale to gently lift the grounded leg to 10°-20° angle. Exhale to lower the lifted leg 10cm from the ground. This is 1 round. Repeat the same for 8-12 counts and change sides.

Awareness: Physical – first to position the body safely on the side, on the leg lifts not to compress the belly and on breathing. Spiritual – on solar plexus (manipura) chakra or sacral (swadhisthana) chakra.

Benefits: Stretches and strengthens the genital area, hamstrings, thighs and the sides of the torso. Tones the abdomen muscles and helps improve digestive system. Burns fat in the areas of hips and thighs.

Precautions: Those with knee, neck, wrist or shoulders conditions should avoid this asana. Those with spinal conditions or spondylitis should totally avoid this practice.

Note: Before relaxing to Matsya Kridasana, can incorporate Anantasana and its variations for practicing. When lowering the leg, the move can be continuous up and down, or with a breath break and the leg grounded. On the 90° leg lift, should not raise leg up straight, as there will be extra pressure on the belly. Intention of this asana is firstly to balance the body on leg raise; if leg cannot go as high as 90°, keep it lower to the comfort zone without compromising the balance. Any of the variations can be given as sequence practice with any order.

75. One-Legged King Pigeon Pose – Eka Pada Rajakapotasana

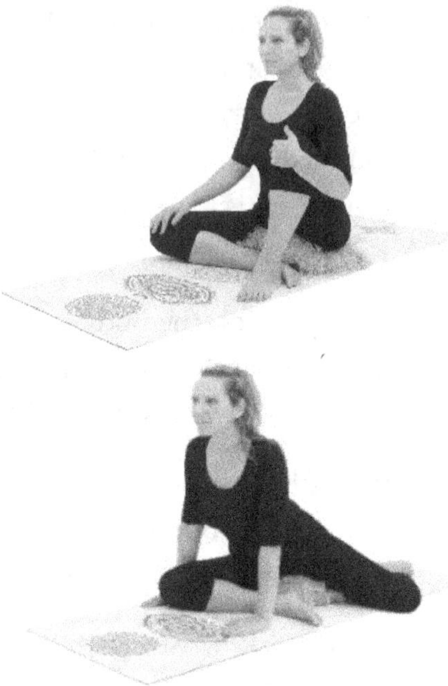

Practice: Sit on a cushion in Sukhasana. Keep the right leg on the ground further away from the perineum to better accommodate the belly and slowly take the left knee up and round it backwards on the floor with the heel close to the hamstring. Adjust the cushion to keep the hip levelled. Inhale to come onto the hands (or fingertips), lengthen the spine, open the chest and on exhalation slowly slide the left leg a little further backwards. [*For some would-be-mums, this may be the limit of their comfort zone; that is fine, do not strain practice*].

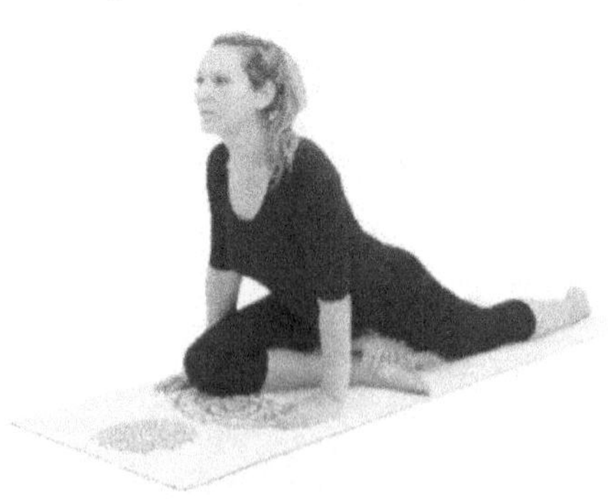

For a flexible would-be-mum, on exhalation, she can very slowly extend the left leg back, with the knee almost straight and the toes rested or pointed to the ground. Adjust the hands and the trunk so the spine is lengthened with the head looking forward to the eyes level. [*For some other would-be-mums, this point may be the limit of their comfort zone; that is fine. The effect of this asana can be felt completely until this point – do not force practice to final stage*].

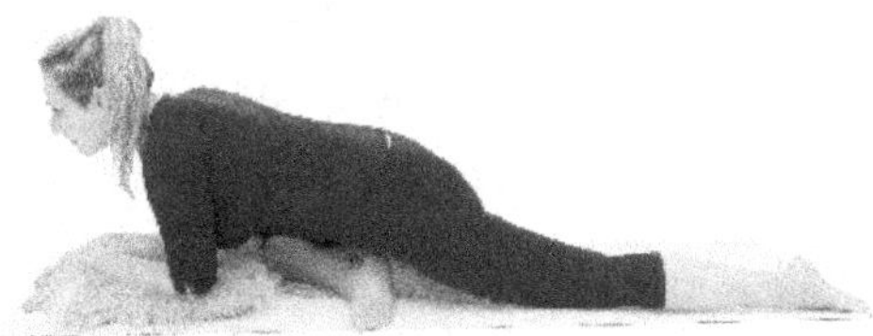

An experienced flexible would-be-mum, needs to make sure her belly is nicely accommodated by taking further away from the perineum the right leg, and if her belly allows her to go further down, on exhalation she can slowly walk down with the help of her palms and either rest the forearms on the ground or on a cushion to help the body lift up so there is no belly compression.

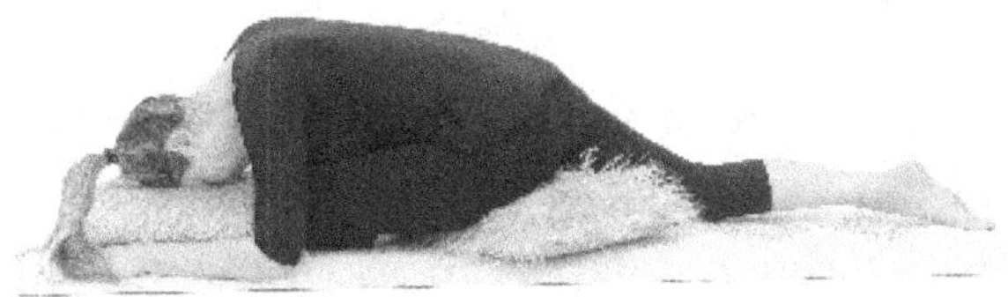

If her body capacity allows her to go even further down, on exhalation she can lower the body to rest the forehead on 1 or 2 cushions to help the body lift up so there is no belly compression and the forearms to be positioned flat on the ground.

To come out of the position, slowly push and walk back with the support of the hands. When the body is up, bend the knee and slowly slide it forward to return to Sukhasana. Repeat the same with the other leg.

Breathing: Inhale to lift knee up. Exhale to slide knee back. Inhale to come onto the hands or fingertips. Exhale to hand walk forward and lower upper body. Normal breathing on final position. Inhale to hand walk backwards and sit up straight the upper body. Normal breathing to adjust body. Exhale to slide knee forward. Normal breathing.

Awareness: Physical – on stretching the neck, shoulders, chest, groin and thighs. Spiritual – on throat (vishuddhi) chakra, sacral (swadhisthana) chakra, root (mooladhara) chakra.

Benefits: It is beneficial to those suffering from sciatica or piriformis syndrome7F[8]. Strengthens the spinal nerves and the back. Increases flexibility and tones up the vertebral column. Stretches the abdomen and pelvis, the hips and the hamstrings. Opens the pelvic region. Opens the chest and improves respiratory system, posture and rounded shoulders – especially in the postnatal period when nursing/breastfeeding the baby. Benefits all the organs and glands between the brain and the thighs.

Precautions: Should be avoided if there is back or pelvic pain. Should not be practiced in the third trimester if it feels uncomfortable. Back bending should be only until the point there is no strain and the breath remains comfortable, as excess bending can contra-indicate during a pregnancy.

Note: Can also be considered a backbend; caution to not overstretch. During pregnancy, from this asana, always come to counter pose in Child's Pose – Shashankasana. During postnatal, can also come to Paschimottanasana. Beginners who never practiced this asana before, may not be able to practice this asana at all during the pregnancy – do not force practice. Even experienced yoga practitioners, while on pregnancy, they may not be able to reach final position – do not force practice. Any practicing must feel comfortable and every would-be-mum should observe her body and its' limitations.

---

[8] The piriformis muscle which is located in the buttock can cause spasm and pain in the buttock area, and that causes the piriformis syndrome. Can also aggravate the sciatic nerve.

76. Lizard Pose – Utthan Pristhasana

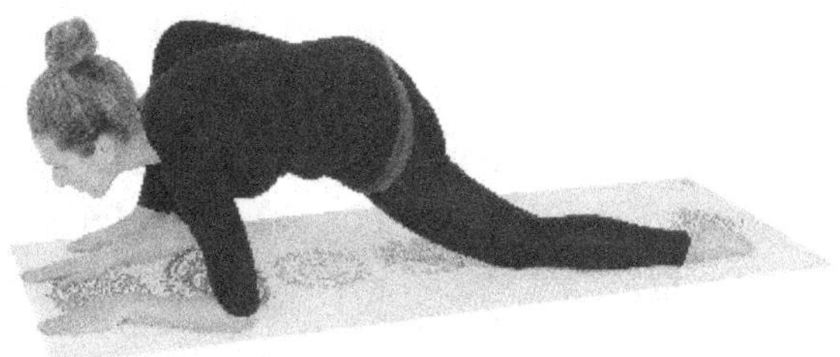

Practice: From Ashwa Sanchalanasana or Bharmanasana, inhale to bring the right knee forward and open sideways to bent at 90° degrees angle. Exhale to slowly extended backwards the left leg to a level there is no tension or jerky movement on the position, particularly in the abdomen area. The hands can be with the palms flat on the floor to the inner side of the right foot, or can be bent by the elbows with lower forearms flat on the ground. To support the hands if on elbows, practitioner can use a cushion underneath to reduce the distance from the ground. Inhale to tilt the head slightly backwards to help a gentle spinal curve, or can look straight with the spine straight. Remain at the position for 3-5 normal breaths. To come out from the position, inhale to bring forward the left knee to rest on the table-top position. Exhale to bring backwards the right bent knee to rest on table-top position, and simultaneously if was on elbows, hand-by-hand come on the palms flat on the ground. Repeat the same with the other leg.

Breathing: Inhale to bend the knee forward. Exhale to extend the leg backward. Normal breathing. Exhale to tilt head back. Normal breathing at the final position. Inhale to return the extended leg to starting position. Exhale to return to starting position the forward bent leg and the hands on table-top position.

Awareness: Physical – on breath control with the movement and not compressing the belly. Spiritual – on solar plexus (manipura) chakra.

Benefits: Opens the hips, pelvis and chest area. Stretches the neck, shoulders, spinal cord and hamstrings. Can relieve from mild back pain. Gives a gentle abdominal stretch and can help constipation. Tones the extended leg.

Precautions: Those with injuries in the areas of hips, knees, ankles, shoulders, elbows, wrists, neck, rib cage or spinal column should avoid this asana. The upper body stretch should not be too deep to avoid hitting the belly on the ground. The extended leg should be extended as far as it feels comfortable. If there is a perineum or symphysis pubic pain this asana should not be practiced.

Note: Can be practiced from second trimester onwards, with all movements to be controlled with awareness on allowing space to the belly. To support the growing belly on third trimester, can increase the distance of the bent knee to the side and use a cushion between the belly and the ground.

Kneeling Asanas & Table-Top Asanas

When on any kneeling position, even for the stronger and fit practitioners, and especially during the second and third trimester it is advisable to always kneel on some support. Can use a folded towel, a soft blanket or fold the mat to ¾ underneath the knees to support the pushing effect on the knees' joint. The knee is the most vulnerable joint during the pregnancy, and since the would-be-mum's weight will start increasing, the knees must be protected when holding the body weight, as well as having support when raising from the knee.

77. Gate Pose – Parighasana

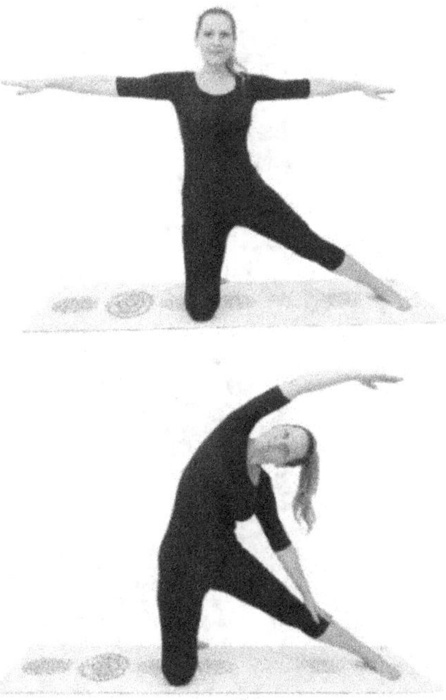

Practice: Sit on the knees with normal breathing until the position is adjusted. Exhale to take the right knee out aligned with the hip joint. Inhale to raise the arms to T-shape with normal breathing until practitioner finds own body center and balance. Can also use the support of a chair of yoga blocks for better stability. Inhale to lift the left arm up, sliding down the right hand on the thigh of the right leg, while bending the upper body to the right side. Side bending limit is the knee or higher. Stay in the position for 2-5 normal breaths with no strain or jerky movement. Inhale to come back to the center. Exhale to gently drop the left arm on a chair or yoga block to maintain balance and safety, or to the sides of the body if it feels comfortable that way. Repeat the same with the right arm and left leg to complete 1 round. Can practice 3-5 rounds.

Modification:

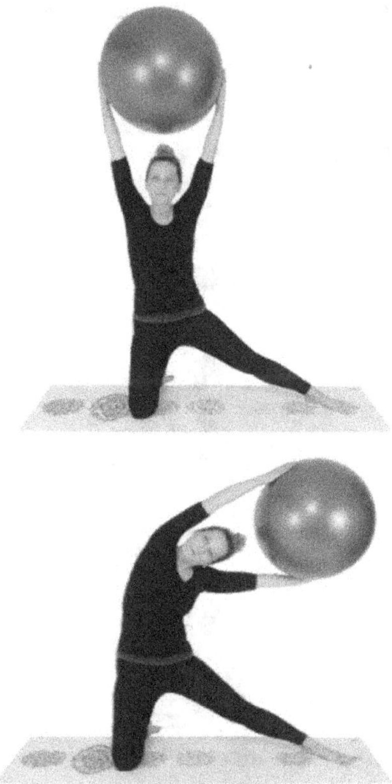

Similarly, this asana can be practiced by holding a Pilates stability ball (55-75cm diameter8F[9]), depending on the height of the practitioner). Sit on

---

[9] **Ball Diameter**   **Height**
    45cm   5' under (≈1.50m)
    55cm   Up to 5'8" (≈1.76m)
    65cm   Up to 6'2" (≈1.88m)
    75cm   Up to 6'7" (≈2.04m)

the knees with normal breathing until the position is adjusted. Keep the Pilates ball positioned in front of the body to help on balancing in the asana. Exhale to take the right knee out aligned with the hip joint. Hold onto the ball and inhale to raise the arms sideways to the right to also side bend the upper body to the right side. Stay in the position for 2-5 normal breaths with no strain or jerky movement. Inhale to come back to the center. Exhale to lower the arms and gently drop the ball in front of the body. Repeat the same with the left leg to complete 1 round. Can practice 3-5 rounds.

Breathing: Normal breathing to find the position. Exhale to take the knee out and extend the leg. Inhale to raise the arm(s). Normal breathing on final position. Exhale to lower arm(s).

Awareness: Physical – on side bending without rounding the spine forward and on breathing. Spiritual – on heart (anahata) chakra, root (mooladhara) chakra and solar plexus (manipura) chakra.

Benefits: It stretches the whole side of the extended leg – hamstring (back of the thigh), groin, adductor (inner thigh), calf muscles, ankle and foot. When balancing on the bent knee, it stretches and strengthens mostly the upper part of the leg – abductor (outer hip), hip flexor (the front of the hip) and quadriceps (thighs). On both the shortened and lengthened side of the torso, it stretches and strengthens the side body, including the abdominal obliques and the muscles along of the spinal column. On the lengthened side also stretches the back muscles. Can increase energy levels.

Precautions: Those with knee conditions should not practice.

Note: Bending should always be on the same side of the extended leg. Avoid rounding the spine forward. Counter poses are Utthita Trikonasana, Kaliasana or Parivritti Janu Sirshasana.

78. Half Camel Pose – Ardha Ushtrasana

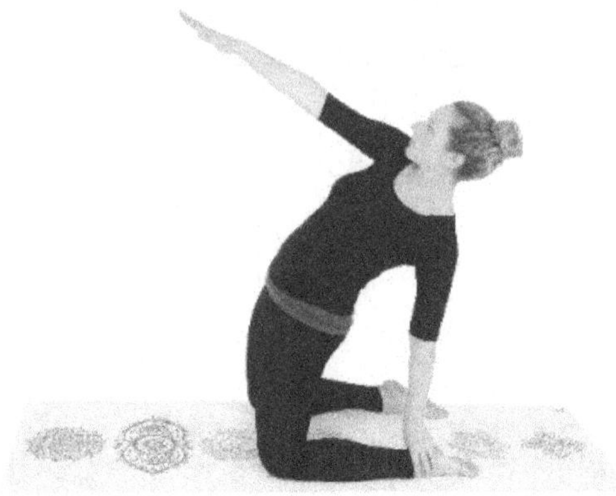

Practice: Sit on Vajrasana and stand on the knees apart with normal breathing until the position feels comfortable – with knees and feet apart to maintain the balance. The toes should be flat on the ground. Sit upright with the trunk straight and breathe normally. This is the starting position.

Inhale to stretch the left arm from sideways and exhale while rotating the movement towards the back to touch the left heel or ankle. Stretch the right arm in front of the head. The head should be slightly tilted backwards and gaze should be fixed at the outstretched hand. Gently push the buttocks forward and the upper body leaning backward. There should be no force on the practice, would-be-mum should listen to her body and bend as little or as much her limit is for comfortable breathing without any jerky movements or strain. Stay in the position for 2-3 normal breaths. Exhale to release the pose by bringing the right hand down and on inhalation slowly bring the left hand forward while uplifting the body to the center. Can repeat the same 3-5 times with normal breathing.

Breathing: Inhale to stretch the left hand to the side. Exhale to touch the left heel or ankle with the left hand. Inhale to raise the right hand. Breathe normally. Exhale to lower the right hand. Inhale to lift up the body to starting position.

Variation 1:

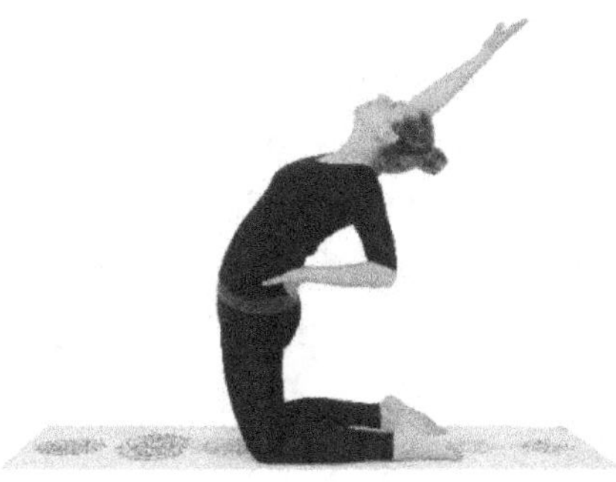

From starting position, place both palms on the hips or lower back. Inhale to raise and stretch the left arm to the back with upper forearm at the same level with the ear. Right hand to remain on the right hip or lower back. Gently push the buttocks forward and the upper body leaning backward. There should be no force on the practice, bend as little or as much for comfortable breathing without any jerky movements or strain. Stay in the final position for 2-3 normal breaths. Exhale to release the pose by bringing the left arm down to the hips or lower back. Inhale and slowly uplift the body to the center. Repeat the same with the right arm to complete 1 round. Can repeat the same for 3-5 rounds with normal breathing on the final position.

Breathing: Inhale to raise and stretch the left arm to the back. Breathe normally at the final position. Exhale to lower the hand. Inhale to lift up the body to starting position.

Variation 2:

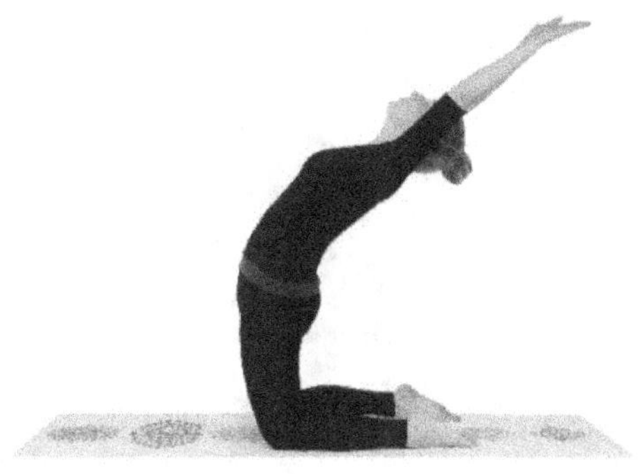

From starting position, place both palms on the hips or lower back. Inhale to raise and stretch one arm at a time to the back with upper forearms at the same level with the ears. Gently push the buttocks forward and the upper body leaning backward. There should be no force on the practice, bend as little or as much for comfortable breathing without any jerky movements or strain. Stay in the final position for 2-3 normal breaths. To release the pose, exhale to bring down to the hips or lower back one arm, inhale and on exhalation bring the other down. Inhale and slowly uplift the body to the center. This is 1 round and can repeat the same for 3-5 rounds with normal breathing on the final position.

Breathing: Inhale to raise the arms to the back. Breathe normally at the final position. Exhale to lower the arms one by one. Inhale to lift up the body to starting position.

Awareness: Physical – on the neck and back stretch and on normal breathing. Spiritual – on heart (anahata) chakra or throat (vishuddhi) chakra.

Benefits: Same as Ushtrasana, but at a reduced level.

Precautions: Those with back or spinal conditions should not practice this asana without the presence of a qualified yoga teacher.

Note: There should be no force on the practice, would-be-mum should listen to her body and bend as little or as much her body limit allows for comfortable breathing without any jerky movements or strain.

79. Camel Pose – Ushtrasana

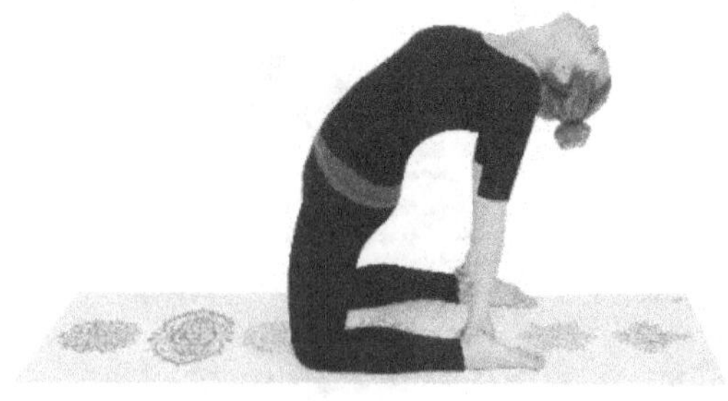

Practice: Sit on Vajrasana and stand on the knees apart with normal breathing until the position feels comfortable – with knees and feet apart to maintain the balance. The toes should be flat on the ground. Sit upright with the trunk straight and breathe normally. Bring both hands behind the hips or on lower back level if that feels comfortable. Find the balance and comfort position while breathing normally. This is the starting position.

Inhale to gently push the hips forward and as the upper body leans backward, with the left hand touch the left heel and with the right hand touch the right heel. The hips should be slightly pushed forward and the head and spine backward until the comfort zone is reached. Stay in the position for 2-3 normal breaths. To come back to the center, slowly release one hand at a time from the heels, bring the head up and lean forward to bring the body to upright position.

Second & Third Trimester

Modification 1:

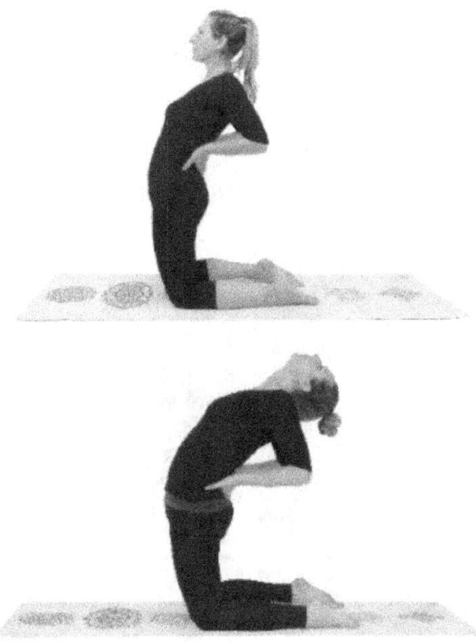

From starting position, inhale to gently push the hips forward and the upper body leans backward. Look up (or straight if still suffering from dizziness and nausea). There should be no force on the practice, would-be-mum should listen to her body and bend as little or as much her body limit allows for comfortable breathing without any jerky movements or strain. Exhale to return to the center.

Modification 2:

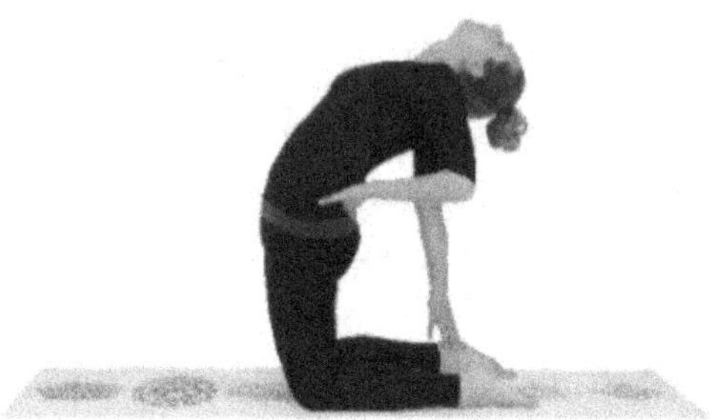

From starting position, inhale to stretch the left arm from sideways and exhale while rotating the movement towards the back to touch the left heel or ankle. The head should be slightly tilted backwards and gaze should be fixed up at the ceiling. Gently push the hips forward with the upper body leaning backward. There should be no force on the practice. Stay in the position for 2-3 normal breaths. Inhale to release the pose and uplift the body to the center and the lowered hand to the hips or lower back. Repeat the same with the other hand to complete 1 round. Can repeat 3-5 rounds with normal breathing.

Modification 3:

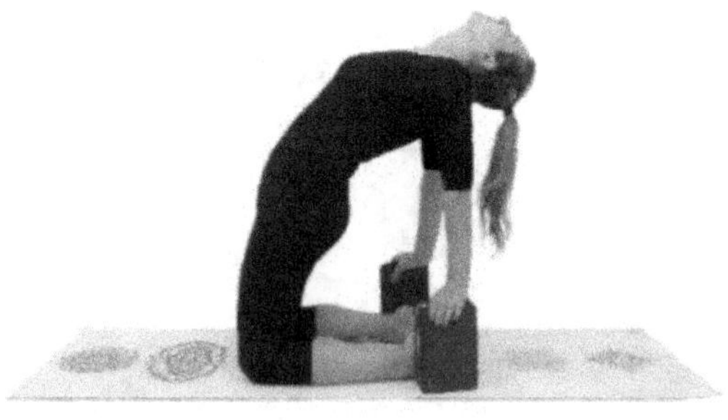

For experienced practitioners on their second trimester onwards who find it difficult to lean backwards to normal Ushtrasana, they can use 2 yoga blocks to allow a good height. Sit on Vajrasana and stand on the knees with normal breathing until the position feels comfortable. The toes should be flat on the ground. Sit upright with the trunk straight. Bring both hands behind the buttocks or on lower back level if that feels comfortable. Find the balance and comfort position while breathing normally. Inhale to gently push the buttocks forward and the upper body leaning backward. When comfortable on this position, place one by one the hands on the yoga blocks to open up the chest and bring the head down by fixing the gaze straight and to the ceiling. Stay in the position for 2-3 normal breaths. Release the pose by bringing the head up and as you are bringing the body to upright position, place one by one the hands to the buttocks or in lower back – what feels comfortable.

Breathing: Normal and soft breathing through the exercise.

Duration: Can practice 2-3 normal breaths on final position. Can repeat up to 3 times.

Awareness: Physical – on throat, spine with normal breathing. Spiritual – on sacral (swadhisthana) chakra or throat (vishuddhi) chakra.

Benefits: This asana is beneficial for the reproductive system during the preconception period. Stimulates the digestive system and stretches the stomach, intestines and prevents constipation. The vertebrae get relaxed with the backward bend and the spinal nerves get stimulated. Can relieve from backache, rounded back and dropping shoulders, and can improve body posture. The thyroid gland gets regulated as the throat and its organs are fully stretched. Since this asana is a chest opener, can benefit respiratory system and expand the lungs – useful for those suffering from asthma and breathlessness in pregnancy. Stretches the abdominal and pelvic region.

Precautions: Those with back or spinal conditions should not practice this asana without the presence of a qualified yoga teacher.

Note: Make sure the body is not over-bending and the back is not curved, especially during the third trimester. There should be no force on the practice, would-be-mum should listen to her body and bend as little or as much her body limit allows for comfortable breathing without any jerky movements or strain. Intention of this modification is to open up the chest and not go all the way down. If the would-be-mum is experienced enough, could maybe be allowed to go all the way down, however, this will be considered as overstretch and she might experience after the practice backache, hip joint pain, knee pain, or rounded ligament pain9F[10]. If we consider baby's health, there is no problem practicing this asana.

From a backward bending asana, it is highly recommended to go to a forward bending one; as a counter-pose, can go to Shashankasana in order to avoid any unnecessary body movement.

80. Table Top Pose – Bharmanasana

From Vajrasana, with the palms of the hands positioned below the shoulder level, tuck the toes or keep them flat on the ground. Keep neutral position of the spine and back. Knees to be separated aligned under the hips during pre-conception, first and fourth trimester. On second and third trimester maintain a gap between the knees to accommodate comfortably the growing belly.

81. Cat and Cow Stretch Pose – Marjariasana

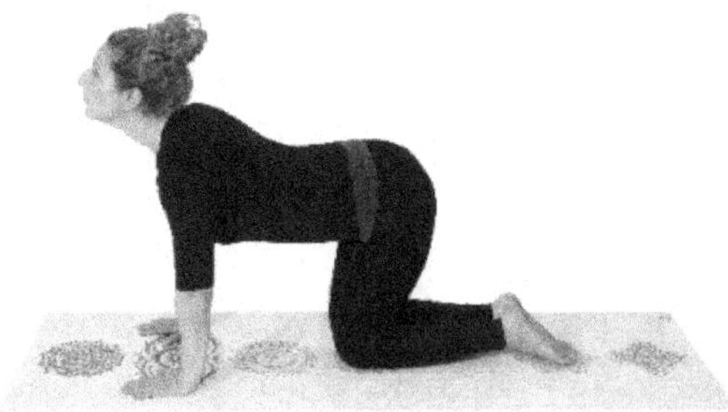

---

[10] It is a common and uncomfortable pain during pregnancy in the abdomen, near the hips or into the groin region.

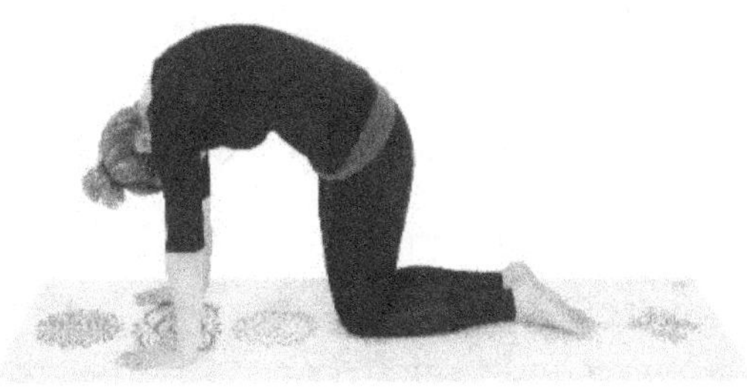

Practice: From Bharmanasana, inhale and slowly come to Cow's pose by tilting the pelvis back while looking up so the back becomes curved in. Exhale and slowly come to Cat's pose by bringing in the chin to the chest and rounding the back. This is 1 round. Can repeat 3-5 rounds or more if needed, with no jerky movement.

Modification 1:

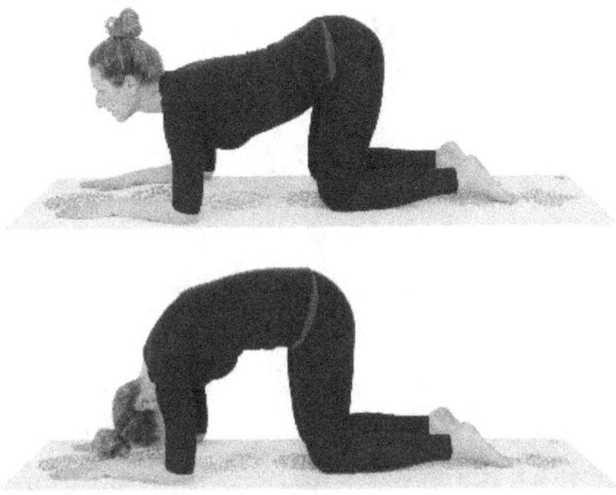

Practice the asanas by coming to table-top position and placing the elbows and the lower arm flat on the ground.

Breathing: Continuous normal breathing with the movement.

Awareness: Physical – stretching the spinal column while synchronizing the breath with the movement. Avoid contraction or overstretch of the abdomen. Spiritual – on sacral (swadhisthana) chakra.

Benefits: Stretches and improves flexibility of the neck, shoulders and spinal column. In the pre-conception phase can tone up the woman's reproductive system and relieve from menstrual cramps.

Note: Especially during the first trimester, where the pregnancy is not yet shown, women tend to overstretch because they are unconscious about their movement. From second trimester onwards, the growing belly makes the would-be-mum more aware of the movement because of the physical grown belly.

82. Thread the Needle Flow – Urdhva Mukha Pasasana Vinyasa

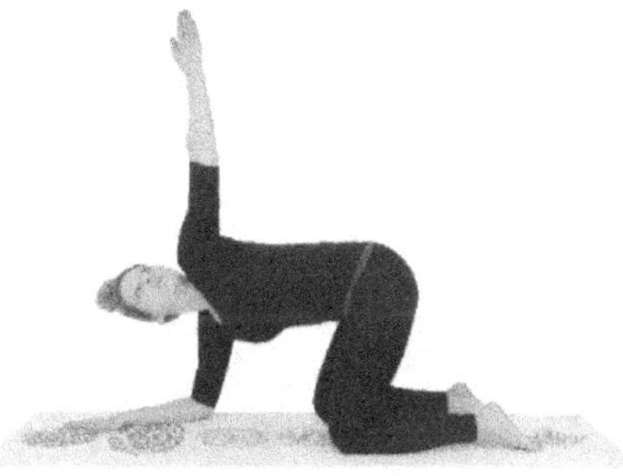

Practice: From Bharmanasana, place the elbows and the lower arm flat on the ground. Inhale to raise right arm up and gently stretch it up to the level there is no overstretch on the belly. Gaze at the extended hand or look straight if still suffering from dizziness and nausea. The hips must be centered without any jerky movement. Stay in the position for 2-3 normal breaths. Exhale to lower the right arm to original position.

Repeat the same with the left arm to complete 1 round. Can practice 3-5 rounds or more if needed.

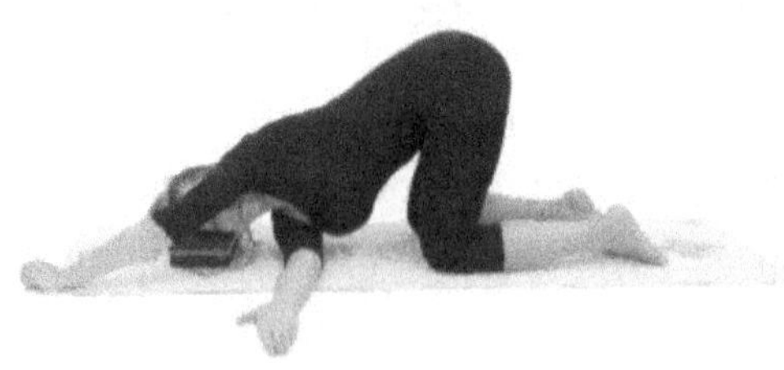

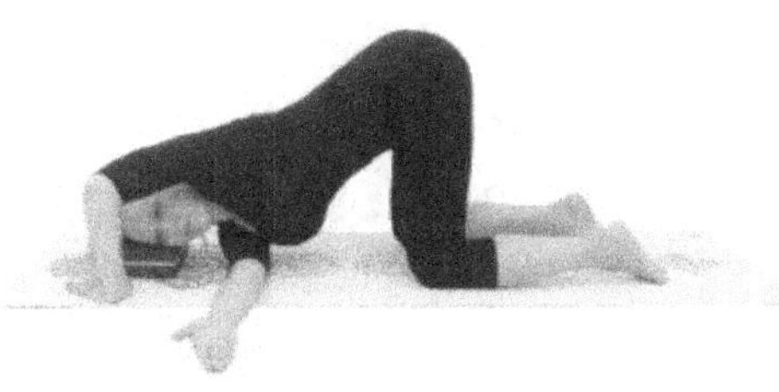

When the arms, shoulders and back is warmed up, inhale to raise up right hand and exhale to twist the hand down on the ground, with upper arm, shoulder joint and ear resting on the ground. For those who find it challenging to bring the shoulder down to the floor, can use a cushion to rest the shoulder and the ear on. For those who find it challenging to keep the ear and the shoulder on the ground, can use a yoga block to rest the ear on. The left hand can either be extended forward or bent at original position. Stay in the position for 2-3 comfortable normal breaths. To come out from the position, return the left hand at original position, push the left palm down, inhale to lift the body up and release to raise the right hand up. Practice one side at a time to avoid any body jerk. Can practice 4-6 times per side, or more if needed.

Variation:

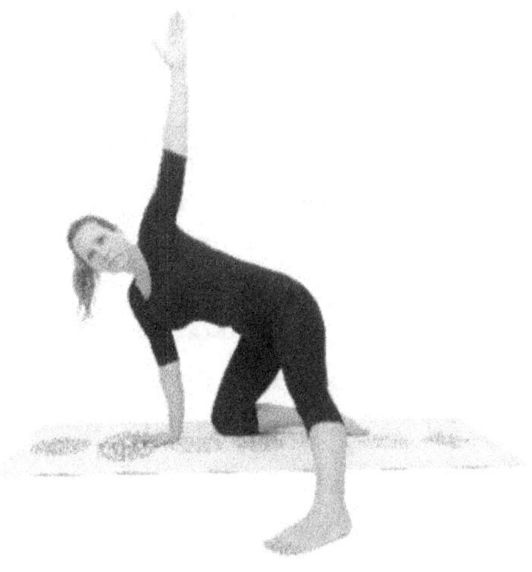

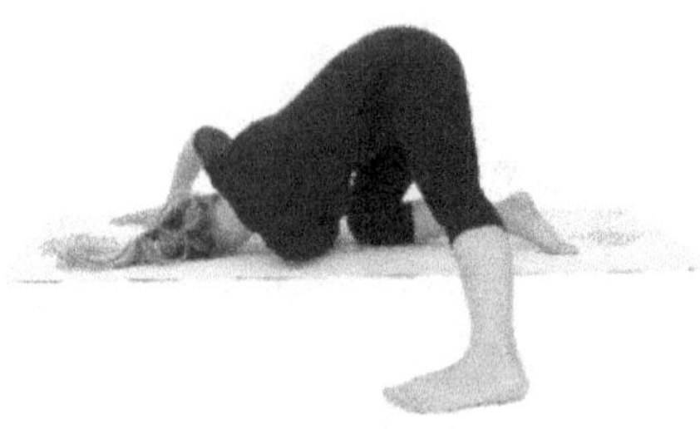

For advanced and experienced practitioners only during the pregnancy, extend the right leg out and sideways, parallel to the hip level. Inhale to raise the right hand up, exhale to bring the right hand down to the ground. To release the pose, inhale to bring the hand up, exhale to rest it on the ground. Inhale to bring the right leg back to original position.

Note: Because of the extended leg and the stretching effect on the inner thigh, it is recommended to use a cushion to rest the shoulder and the ear, so a good height is maintained for the twist.

Breathing: Inhale to raise the arm. Normal breath on final position. Exhale to lower the arm and/or rest the shoulder and ear on the ground. Normal breathing on final position. Inhale to lift the body up to release the pose.

Awareness: Physical – on stretching the arms and shoulders, the lower and middle back. Spiritual – on sacral (swadhisthana) chakra or solar plexus (manipura) chakra.

Benefits: The twisted asanas massage the internal organs and also help to release body toxins. Stretches the side of the body, the neck, shoulders, arms and upper back. Opens up the chest area and helps respiratory system.

Precautions: Those with neck, shoulders, spine, back or knees conditions should avoid practicing. If vinyasa makes would-be-mum breathless on the final position, can use a support system to increase the height from the ground and the rested parts, and if still challenging, should abort practice.

Note: Stretch the arm up only to the level it feels comfortable to breathe and there is no overstretch on the belly. Keep the knees wider open and use a support system under them such as a folded blanket to take excess pressure from knee joints. The hands can be slightly forward from the shoulder level to allow a comfortable extended gap between the knees and the hands for the crossing of the hand so the belly does not get compressed. Use a cushion to support the head and the shoulder to give the extra height to the body to allow movement without compressing the belly to the ground. Adjust the body positioning to feel comfortable. It is a great asana for the second trimester to stretch the whole body, as well as for the postnatal duration to release tension from bad body posture. Not to be practiced on third trimester.

83. Bird Dog or Balancing Table Top Pose – Parsva Balasana

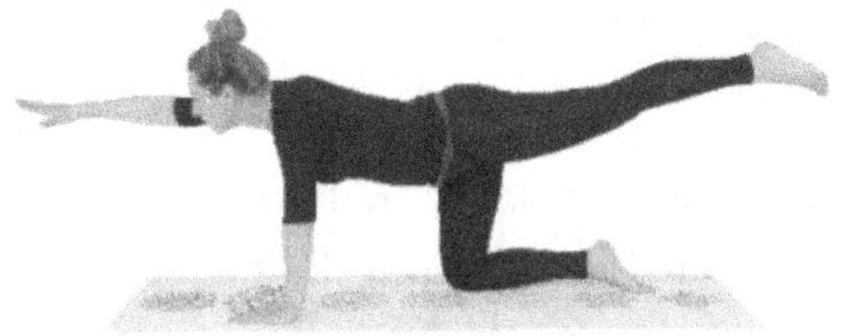

Practice: From Bharmanasana, inhale to extend the right leg back and parallel to the hip level. Find the balance with normal breathing and inhale to extend the left hand in front of the head parallel to the shoulder level. Stay for 1-2 breaths. Can either gaze at the extended hand or gaze down with neck and spine aligned. Slowly bring the left hand to the ground and then lower the right leg to bring the knee to the ground. Repeat the same for 6-8 counts on the same leg. When ready, repeat the same with the other leg. This is 1 round and can practice 3-5 rounds.

Modification 1: If would-be-mum is experienced in practicing and can maintain balance with no strain, can practice with alternate movement of opposite arm, opposite leg for 12 total counts to complete 1 round. Normal breathing on bharmanasana. Can repeat for 3 rounds total.

Modification 2: Can practice the same with the support of a chair to rest the extended hand if balance needs to be maintained. When using a chair as a support system, can stay in the position for 3-5 normal breaths before changing sides.

Breathing: Normal breathing on starting and finishing position. Inhale to extend the leg back. Inhale to extend the hand forward. Exhale to lower the leg. Exhale to lower the hand.

Awareness: Physical – on extending opposite leg, opposite arm. Spiritual – on sacral (swadhisthana) chakra or root (mooladhara) chakra.

Benefits: Stretches and tones up the arms and shoulders, core, gluteal, hips, thighs and knees muscles. Opens the chest area and improve respiratory system. Opens the hips, helps on balance and flexibility. Strengthens the spinal nerves, which can help relax the sciatica nerves. Tightens the muscles around the vagina and can be practiced for its effects in the postnatal duration.

Precautions: Those with knee, wrist, ankle or wrist injuries and those with spinal or back conditions should avoid the practice. One must be aware of the neck and not to overarch the lower back, especially if there is excess curve in lumbar.

Note: Some women have the feeling in that practice that the core is engaged and the abdomen muscles are pulling up, similar to having a contraction effect. In such case, it is advisable for them to practice with a chair and close to a wall. When the leg gets extended backwards, the sole of the foot rests to the wall, and when the hand gets extended forward it rests on the chair. By that way, there will be no core engagement.

84. Donkey Kicks Straight Raised Leg

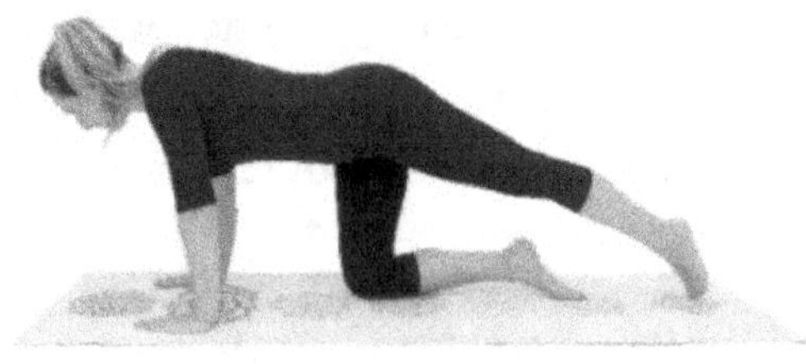

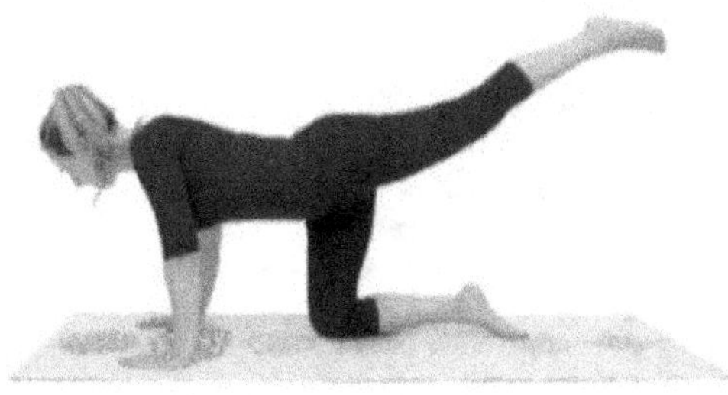

Practice: From Bharmanasana, inhale to extend one leg back with the toes tuck on the ground. Press the toes, and with continuous breathing gently push the hip backwards and forward to feel the stretch on the cuff muscle and hamstring. Can practice this 3-5 times back and forward per leg. When practitioner is warmed-up, inhale to lift the leg up parallel to the hip level or higher. Exhale to slowly lower the leg down to the ground. Continue practice on same leg for 10-15 counts. Repeat the same with the other leg.

Breathing: Normal breathing on starting and finishing position. Inhale to extend the leg back. Inhale to raise the leg up. Exhale to lower the leg.

Awareness: Physical – on keeping the neck and the spine aligned, balance and breathing. Spiritual – on solar plexus (manipura) chakra, sacral (swadhisthana) chakra or root (mooladhara) chakra.

Benefits: Stretches and tones up the arms and shoulders, core, gluteal, hips, thighs and knees muscles. Opens the chest area and improve respiratory system. Opens the hips, helps on balance and flexibility. Strengthens the spinal nerves, which can help relax the sciatica nerves. Tightens the muscles around the vagina and can be practiced for its effects in the postnatal duration.

Precautions: Those with knee, wrist, ankle or wrist injuries and those with spinal or back conditions should avoid the practice. One must be aware of the neck and not to overarch the lower back, especially if there is excess curve in lumbar.

85. Dog Pose – Shvanasana

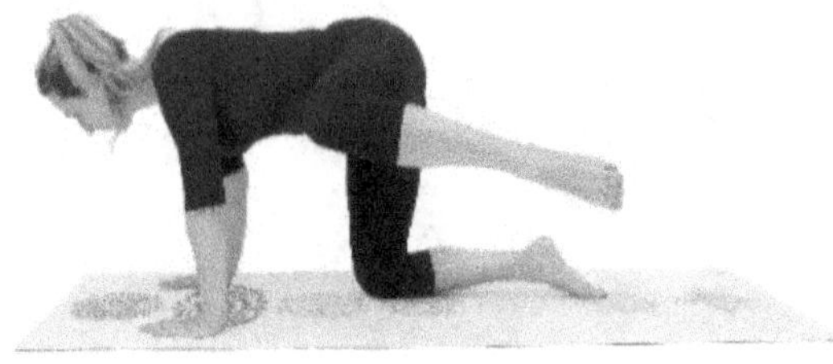

Practice: From Bharmanasana inhale to lift the left leg sideways by maintain the knee bent. Exhale to return the leg to the center. Repeat the same 10-15 times per leg.

Breathing: Inhale to side lift the leg. Exhale to lower. Breathing and movement should be controlled and continuous.

Awareness: Physical – on synchronized breathing with the movements. Spiritual – sacral (swadhisthana) chakra.

Benefits: Stretches the neck, arms, shoulders, elbows, wrists, chest, back, hips, quadriceps, hamstrings and knees. Strengthens and tones the shoulders, glutes and adductor muscles.

Precautions: Those with imbalanced blood pressure and injuries in the arms, shoulders, wrists, back, hips and knees should avoid this asana.

Note: Can be practiced during the second and third trimester to open up the pelvis, but movement must be controlled when balancing on one leg with no strain or jerky movements.

Standing and Balancing Asanas

As an extra precaution, whenever there is a practitioner wearing glasses, it is recommended to always have the support of a wall or a chair on standing and balancing asanas.

86. Palm Tree Pose – Tadasana

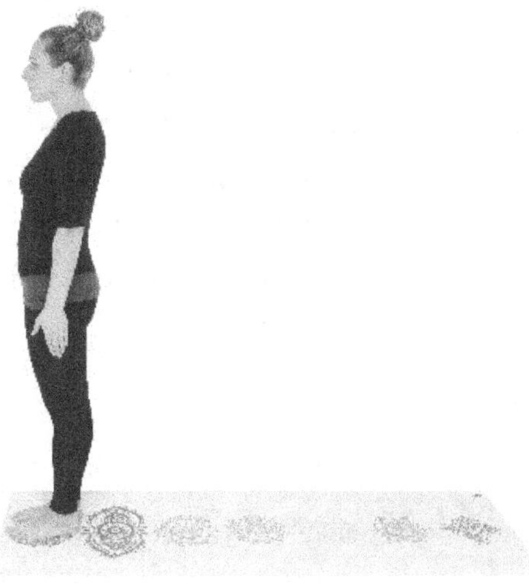

Practice: It is a basic standing pose with the feet apart about 10cm and the spine erect. The hands are parallel to the sides of the body, with the palms facing or touching the sides of the glutes. With normal breathing, distribute the body weight equally on both feet. Fix the gaze at a point slightly above the head level. The classic form of this asana requires interlocked hands and arms raised above the head, which practice will be safer with the support of a wall on the back. In this modification, keep the hands parallel to the sides of the body or inhale to raise the hands in front of the body with palms facing the ground or gently touching a wall. Exhale to hold the position of the hands. Inhale to come on the toes. Exhale to lower the heels to the ground. Hold the position on the toes for 2 normal breaths before lowering the heels to take another 2 normal breaths. This is 1 round. Can practice 10 rounds. Repeat the same for another 10 rounds, but this time on slow and continuous speed up and down.

Breathing: Inhale on upward movement. Exhale on downward movement. Normal breathing when holding the position.

Awareness: Physical – on breathing, balance and strengthening of lower limb. Spiritual – on sacral (swadhisthana) chakra or root (mooladhara) chakra to maintain balance and then to third-eye (ajna) chakra.

Benefits: Helps mind and body balance. Improves the body posture and relaxes and tones the body muscles. By stretching the spine on its classical form of practice, the spinal nerves get relaxed. It is said that if practiced frequently, especially from kids, it helps to increase the height of the practitioner, as it enables the bones to grow longer. During the first and second trimester tones the abdominal muscles and nerves and also stretches the intestines. The modification mainly focuses on engaging the glutes and strengthening the whole lower limb muscles.

Precautions: Since it is a standing asana and may be required to stand for some time, those with recent surgery or conditions in the areas of knees, hips or spine should not practice.

87. Swaying Palm Tree Pose – Tiryak Tadasana

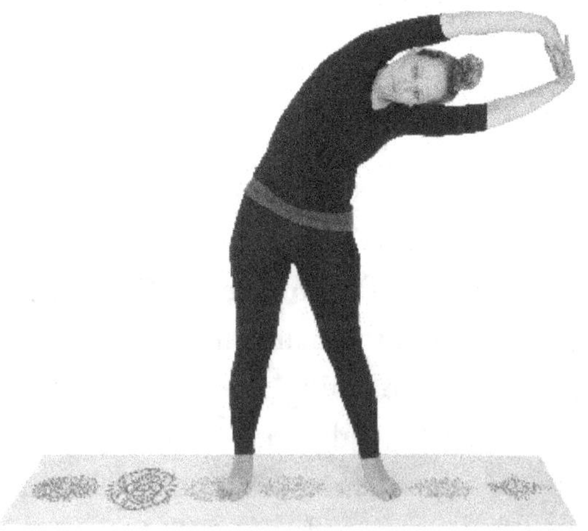

Practice: With the feet hips apart and the spine erect, inhale to stretch the arms above the head and interlock the hands with palms facing the ceiling, where simultaneously the shoulders and chest should be also stretched. Exhale to bend and outstretch the trunk to the right side until the point practitioner feels comfortable. Inhale to return to the center. Exhale to bend and outstretch the trunk to the left side with the arms always outstretched above the head. This is 1 round. Can practice 5 rounds.

Awareness: Physical – on synchronization of breath and controlled, slow and continuous movement to come in and out of the position; on maintaining the arms' alignment above the head during the practice and keeping them still; trunk remains erect and still. Spiritual – on solar plexus (manipura) chakra or heart (anahata) chakra.

Benefits: Stretches, strengthens and lengthens the rib cage and the muscles in the areas of hips, middle back, arms and shoulders. Tones the glutes if during the practice these are engaged.

Precautions: Those with hip joint, ankle or shoulder conditions should avoid the practice.

88. Standing Spinal Twist Pose – Katichakrasana

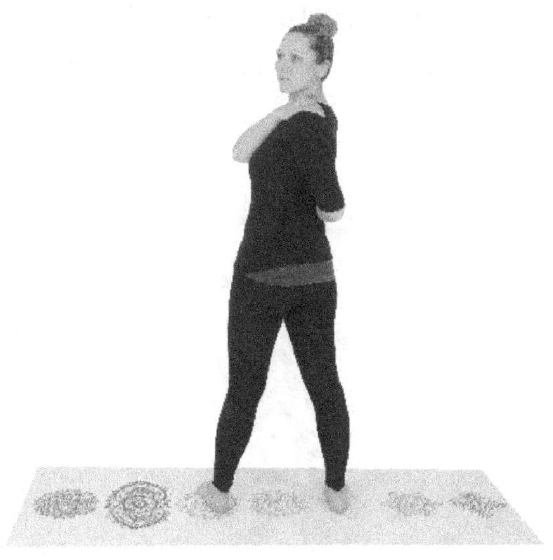

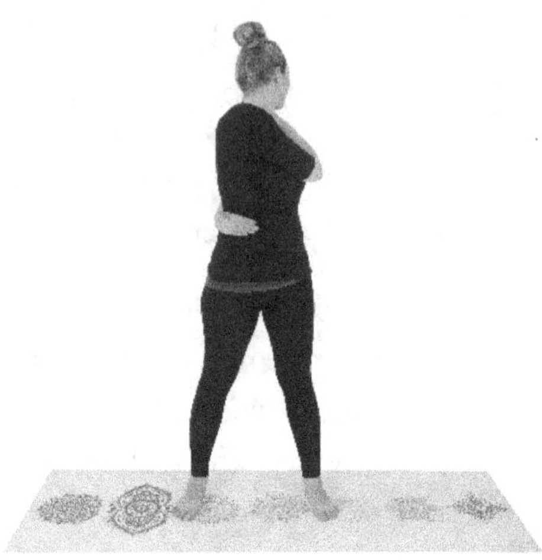

Practice: Begin in Tadasana with the arms in front of the torso and twist from left to right and vice versa. The lower body remains still; the upper body is only moving. Engage your core and hips throughout the practice. Inhale to twist to the left and at the same time place the right palm of the hand on the left shoulder and the left hand by the waist. Stay in that position for 2-3 breaths. Exhale to twist deeper. Inhale to exhale to the right and place the left palm of the hand on the right shoulder and the right hand by the waist. Stay in that position for 2-3 breaths. Exhale to twist deeper. This is 1 round. Can practice 5-10 rounds.

Variation 1:

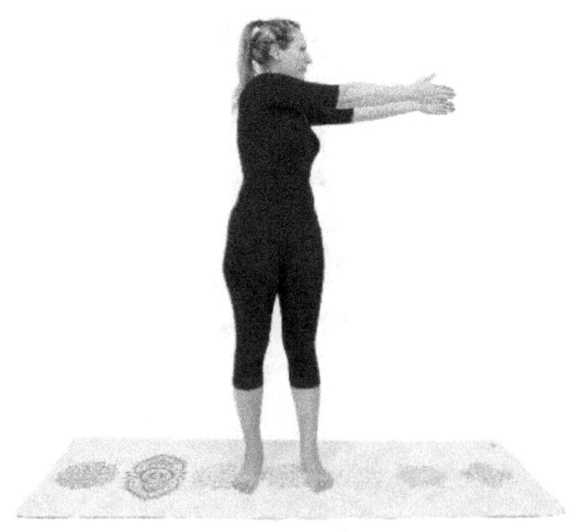

Outstretch the arms in front of the torso with the palms facing each other. The lower body remains still; the upper body is only moving. Engage your core and hips throughout the practice. Inhale to twist to the left where the outstretched arms follow the motion to the left. Stay in the position for 2-3 breaths and exhale to the right to repeat the same. This is 1 round. Can practice 5-10 rounds.

Variation 2: With the Baby

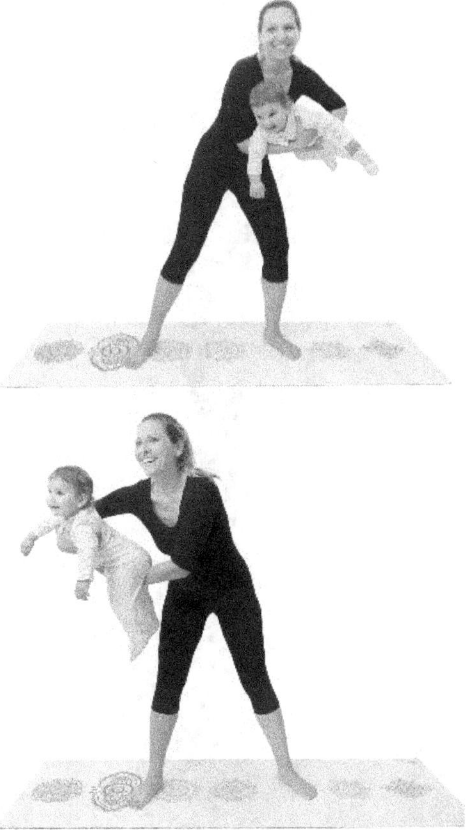

Grasp the baby with safety close to your torso. Open the legs to adjust balance and stability to personal comfort level. Slightly lean torso forward, extend the arms in front of the torso to comfort level and twist from side to side. Baby's weight works as weight lifting exercise and tones and strengthens the whole upper body. Be cautious, the movement shall be done by the waist to avoid any lower back injury.

Awareness: Physical – on synchronization of breath and controlled, slow and continuous movement to come in and out of the position. Spiritual – on solar plexus (manipura) chakra or heart (anahata) chakra.

Benefits: Stretches and strengthens the rib cage and the muscles in the areas of middle back, arms and shoulders. Tones the glutes if during the practice these are engaged.

Precautions: Those with arms or shoulders conditions should avoid the practice.

89. Airplane Pose – Kati Sakti Vikasaka

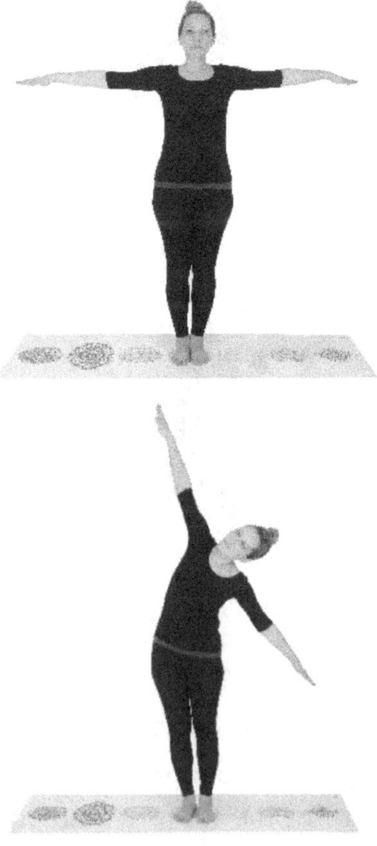

Practice: Begin with the feet together (or slightly apart from second trimester onwards) and spine erect, inhale to outstretch the arms sideways into a T-shape. By maintaining the T-shape on the arms, exhale to bend and outstretch the trunk to the right side until the point practitioner feels comfortable; aim to touch the calf. Inhale to return to the center. Exhale to bend and outstretch the trunk to the left side. This is 1 round. Practice 5-10 rounds.

Awareness: Physical – on synchronization of breath and controlled, slow and continuous movement to come in and out of the position; on maintaining the arms' alignment during the practice and keeping them still; trunk remains erect and still. Spiritual – on solar plexus (manipura) chakra or heart (anahata) chakra.

Benefits: Stretches, strengthens and lengthens the rib cage and the muscles in the areas of hips, middle back, arms and shoulders. Tones the glutes if during the practice these are engaged.

Precautions: Those with hip joint, ankle or shoulder conditions should avoid the practice.

90. One-Legged Prayer or Tree Pose – Eka Pada Pranamasana

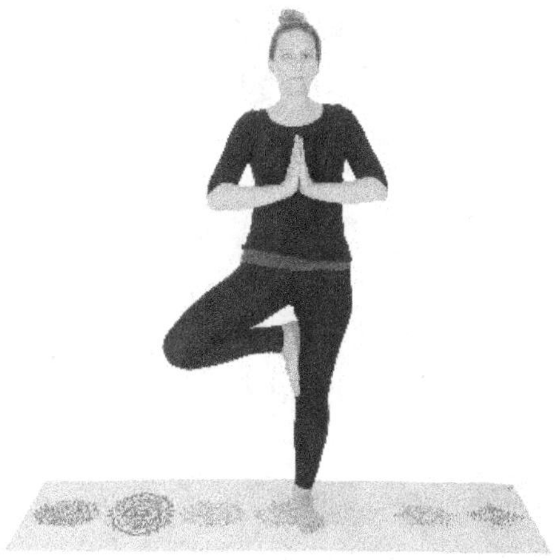

Practice: By standing upright and the feet together or slightly apart bring the arms to the sides of the body. In this initial position, take a few breaths, relax and fix the gaze at any eye level point to find your balance. Slowly adjust the body weight equally to both legs, and slowly shift the body weight to the left leg. Lift up the right heel, rest it above the ankle with the toes still touching the ground. Maintain the balance and slowly slide up the right foot to rest the sole of the foot in the inner thigh of the left leg. Maintain the gaze fixed during the practice in order to have better balance. When the body is balanced and comfortable, slowly inhale and bring both hands to Namaste Mudra in front of the chest. Stay in the final position for a few breaths and slowly exhale to release the hands and then slowly slide down the leg. Repeat the same by shifting the body weight to the other leg.

Variation 1:

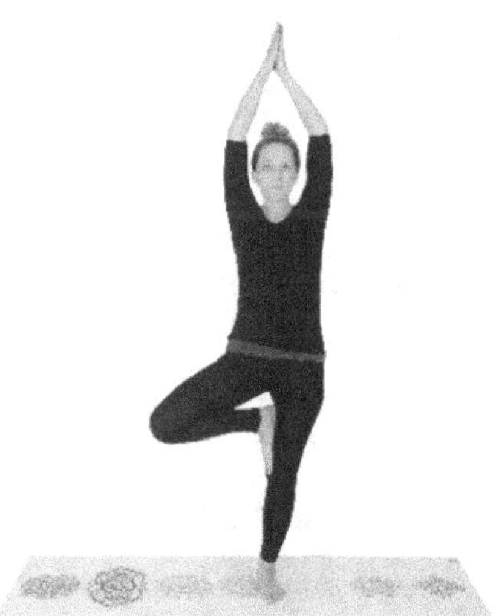

When the body is balanced and comfortable, slowly inhale and raise the arms above the head with palms together.

Variation 2: With the Baby

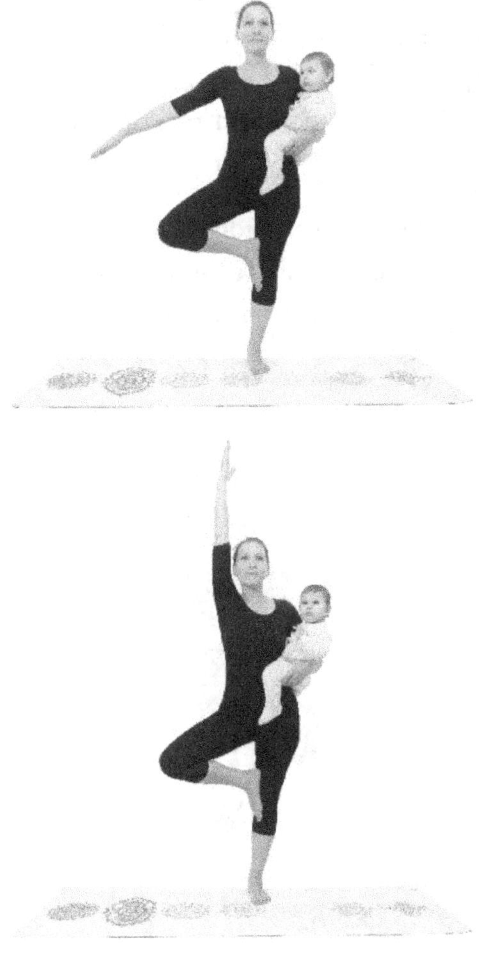

During the fourth trimester and through the first few years of motherhood, can practice Eka Pada Pranamasana by holding the baby to your sides. Physical benefits of practicing with the baby is to increase strength to maximum, depending the baby's weight as it grows, as well as tone up the whole body. Especially the non-experienced practitioners should always practice with the support of a wall or chair for safety reasons. To maintain the balance, the gaze must be fixed at any eye level point and the sole of the foot to be positioned close to the knee area — the closest the sole of the foot is on the perineum, the more demanding the pose becomes. A lot of strength is required in the lower limb, the core must be engaged to maintain the balance, the spine must be erect and the baby must be safely hold onto. Beginners can try to raise the hand diagonally open and parallel to the thigh of the bent leg to help balancing. Intermediate and advanced practitioners can raise one hand above the head.

When practicing with the baby, duration is relative. Baby may be moving, in which case it is recommended to abort this practice. If baby is cooperating, can hold on the final position for up to 1 or 2 minutes, with or without support.

Modification 1:

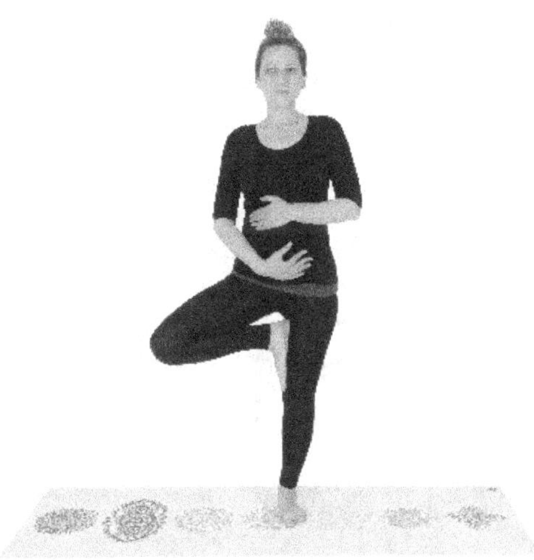

When the body is balanced and comfortable, slowly inhale and nicely bring both palms to hug the belly. Can practice this throughout the whole pregnancy to also connect with the unborn baby.

Modification 2:

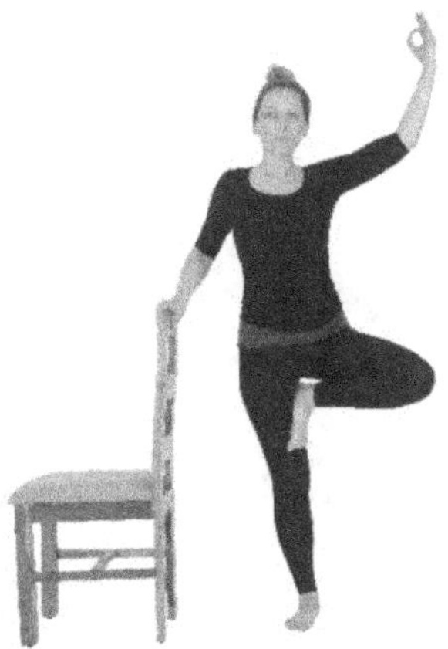

In the final position, it is recommended to hold onto a chair to maintain the balance. When the body is balanced and comfortable, slowly inhale and bring the right hand up while the left hand is holding into the chair. When and if you feel comfortably balanced, may slowly bring the other hand up. Stay in the final position for a few breaths and slowly exhale to release the hands one-by-one and then slide down the leg. Repeat the same by shifting the body weight to the other leg.

Breathing: Normal breathing.

Duration: Practice up to 3 rounds per leg, holding the final position for maximum 10-15 seconds, or with support maximum 30 seconds.

Awareness: Physical – fixing the gaze at eye level. Spiritual – on eyebrow center (ajna) chakra or heart (anahata) chakra.

Benefits: Strengthens the leg, ankle and foot muscles. Opens the pelvic region. Improves balance and coordination between mind and body. Stimulates the nervous system.

Precautions: Those suffering from ankle and/or knee conditions should avoid this asana.

Note: The same variations and modifications can be practiced through all four trimesters.

91. Triangle Pose – Trikonasana

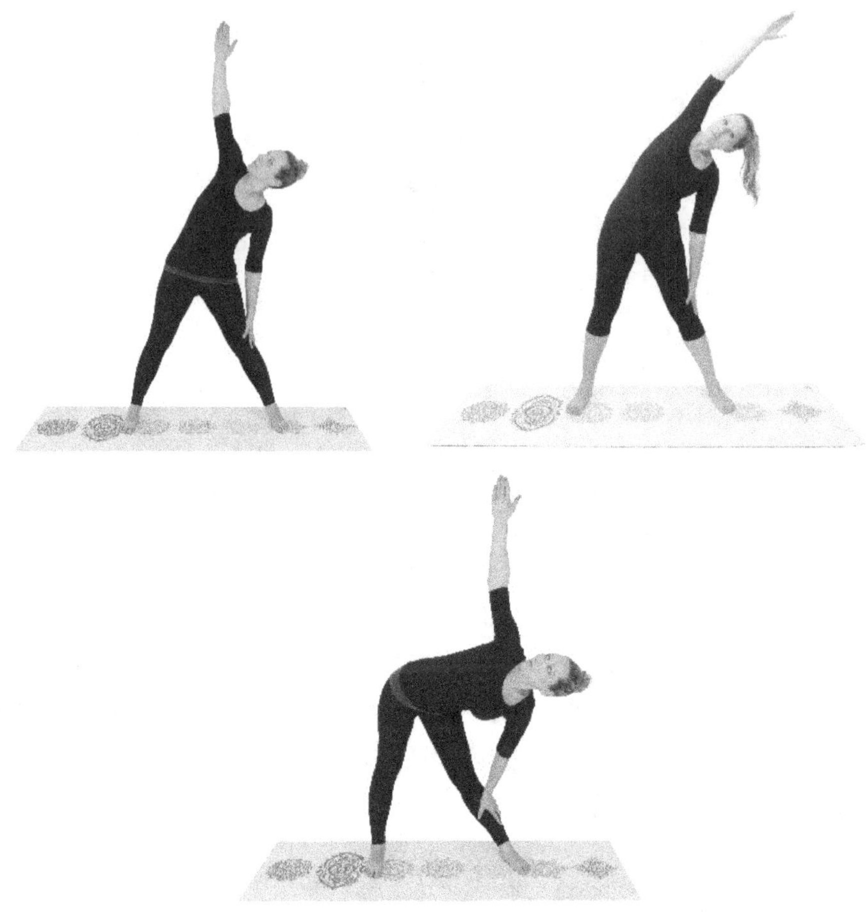

Practice: During the first trimester, the legs should be spread as much as it is the width of the yoga mat and keep straight. In the second and third trimester the legs can be spread open wider and can slightly bend the knee of the same side of the bending. The leg positioning should be right foot opening on 90° degrees to the right side and the left foot should be on 45° degrees on diagonal position. Inhale to raise the arms open sideways to shoulder level so they are in straight line and parallel to the ground. Avoid any compression in the abdomen area. This is the starting position. Exhale to bend to the right from the hips by maintaining the arms stretched to follow the bent movement. The right hand may come only until the shin bone, or above the knee, which is OK. The would-be-mums should go down to whichever extent feels comfortable, without any stain. During the first trimester, look forward when in the final position, to avoid any dizziness. During the second and third trimester, look up at the left hand when in the final position. Inhale to come up to starting position with the arms in straight line. Exhale to shift to the other side and repeat the same with the other leg to complete 1 round. Can practice 5-10 rounds.

Variation:

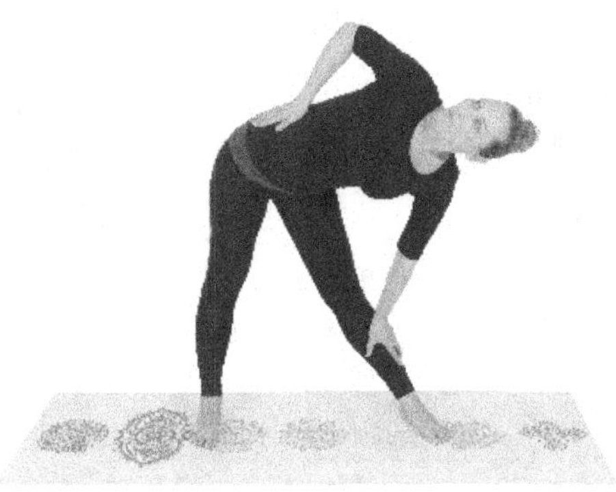

Those who experience difficulties to balance with the arm outstretched, suffer from severe dizziness or light back pain can bend and hold the knee or shin bone with the same side hand and the other hand can be positioned by the waist line.

Breathing: Inhale to raise the arms. Exhale to bend. Normal breathing on final position. Inhale to come up to starting position.

Awareness: Physical – stretching the trunk, legs and arms, maintaining the balance and on controlled breathing with the movement.

Benefits: Opens up and stretches the whole chest area and the abdomen sides; can be helpful to create more space in the rib cage. Opens up the upper back and can relieve from pain in the upper back area. Tones up and opens the pelvic region. Stretches the inner thighs. Strengthens the leg muscles and loosens the hips and knees. Improves balance.

Precautions: Should avoid practice if suffering from strong back pain or pelvic pain; prolapsed uterus or complicated pregnancy.

Note: Bending should be sideways and not forward. In the second and third trimester when the distance of the feet can be increased, the inner thigh muscles and the top of the thighs are getting stretched.

92. Extended Triangle Pose – Utthita Trikonasana

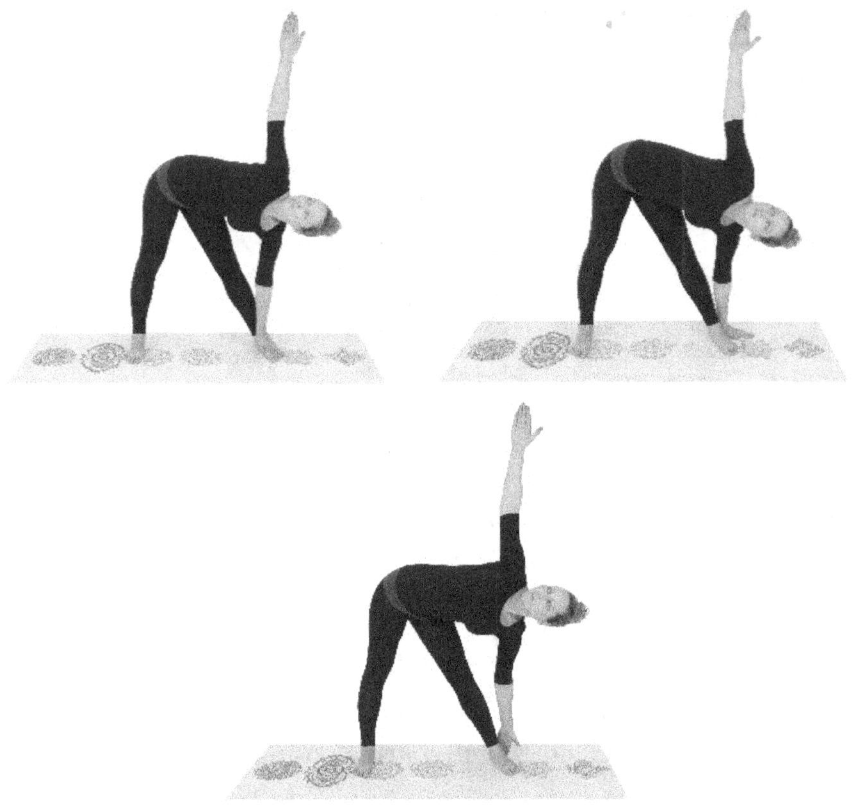

Practice: From Samasthiti, open the feet approximately 4 feet ≈ 1,2 m and extend the arms in a T-shape position with the palms facing downwards. Stretch the arms to opposite direction to feel the chest expanding. The feet should be positioned in a way the body is comfortable for the side bend, however, it is recommended to attempt to turn the left foot out to 90° degrees and the right foot slightly inwards or facing straight in front of the body. Exhale to side bend from the spine by keeping the torso sides equally stretched on the hands T-shape positioning. The right heel should be pressed on the ground while bending. The palm of the lowered hand can be on top of the foot or on the side of the foot or touch the heel with the fingers. Stay in that position for 3-5 normal breaths.

Breathing: Exhale to side bend. Normal breathing at final position.

Awareness: Physical – on breathing, side bend movement and muscles engagement. Spiritual on heart (anahata) chakra, root (mooladhara) chakra or sacral (swadhisthana) chakra.

Benefits: Increases stability. Stretches and flexes the spinal cord and rib cage. Opens the hips and shoulders. Helps to reduce stress and anxiety.

Precautions: Avoid this asana if suffering from imbalanced blood pressure, neck, spinal, back or leg injuries.

Note: A yoga block to support smaller side bending can be used for palm or fingers to touch. The legs should be straight during the practice and the muscles engaged.

93. Extended Side Angle Pose – Utthita Parsvakonasana

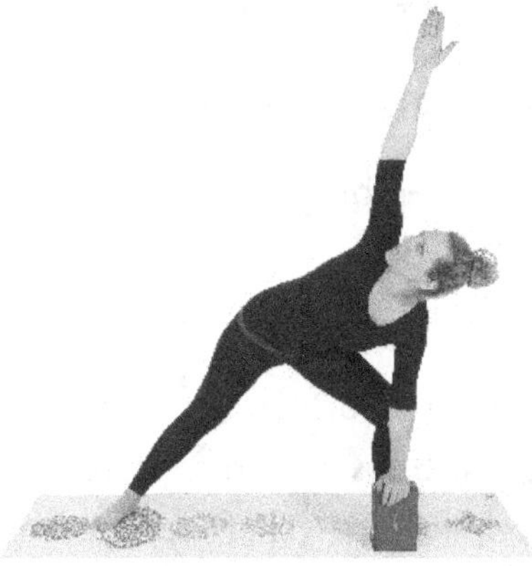

Practice: From Samasthiti, open the feet approximately 4 feet ≈ 1,2 m and extend the arms in a T-shape position with the palms facing downwards. Stretch the arms to opposite direction to feel the chest expanding. The feet should be positioned in a way the body is comfortable for the side bend, however, it is recommended to attempt to turn the left foot out to 90° degrees and the right foot slightly inwards or facing straight in front of the body. Side bend from the spine by keeping the torso sides equally stretched on the hands T-shape positioning. The right heel should be pressed on the ground while bending the left knee to a 90° degree angle. Attempt to have the left thigh parallel to the ground only closer to the end of third trimester and after physical body has totally recovered from childbirth. In all other phases of pregnancy, the left thigh should be adjusted higher to avoid effects similar to Squatting Asanas. To achieve the balance in that position and a strong posture, use the support of a yoga block to hold on with the left hand. The left arm should be aligned with the shin; and the right arm with the palm facing downwards should be raised over the right ear. Fix the gaze at the right palm or fingers and press the right hip towards the ground. Remain at the final position for 3-5 normal breaths. Inhale to slowly release the pose by bringing the hands and torso to original position first, then straighten the left leg. Switch sides to repeat the same with the other leg.

Variation: Can practice the same by resting and pressing down the left forearm on the left thigh of the bent knee. The forearm should be pressed down to prevent left shoulder from lifting up and aggravating the neck.

Breathing: Normal breathing at final position.

Awareness: Physical – on breathing and body alignment understanding to stretch the whole body. Spiritual – on heart (anahata) chakra, sacral (swadhisthana) chakra or root (mooladhara) chakra.

Benefits: Is a restorative pose for flat feet and sciatica. Stimulates the abdominal area and organs. Boosts energy. Stretches and flexes the spine, back and legs side muscles, helps relief from lower backache, therefore improves body posture and should be practiced more by those who have a sitting job. Strengthens the whole lower limb (inner thighs, calves, knees, ankles and toes. Regular practice can help with chronic constipation issues and also strengthen the skeletal system.

Precautions: It is an advanced asana and beginners first introduced to yoga during pregnancy should avoid this practice as it could irritate the joints.

Those with neck injury or pain, should avoid gazing the extended arm. Avoid this asana if suffering from high blood pressure or neck, shoulders, hips or knees conditions.

Note: If fixing the gaze at the right palm or fingers at the final position causes dizziness or imbalance, can fix the gaze looking forward. By bending one knee and extended opposite leg, the practitioner flexes the inner thighs, stretches the gluteal muscles while strengthens the outer leg muscles and tones the hips. This asana can be given as a slow and steady vinyasa with Trikonasana, Virabhadrasana II, Viparita Virabhadrasana and Parighasana, with counter poses Ardha Uttanasana and Ardha Chandrasana.

94. Warrior I – Virabhadrasana I

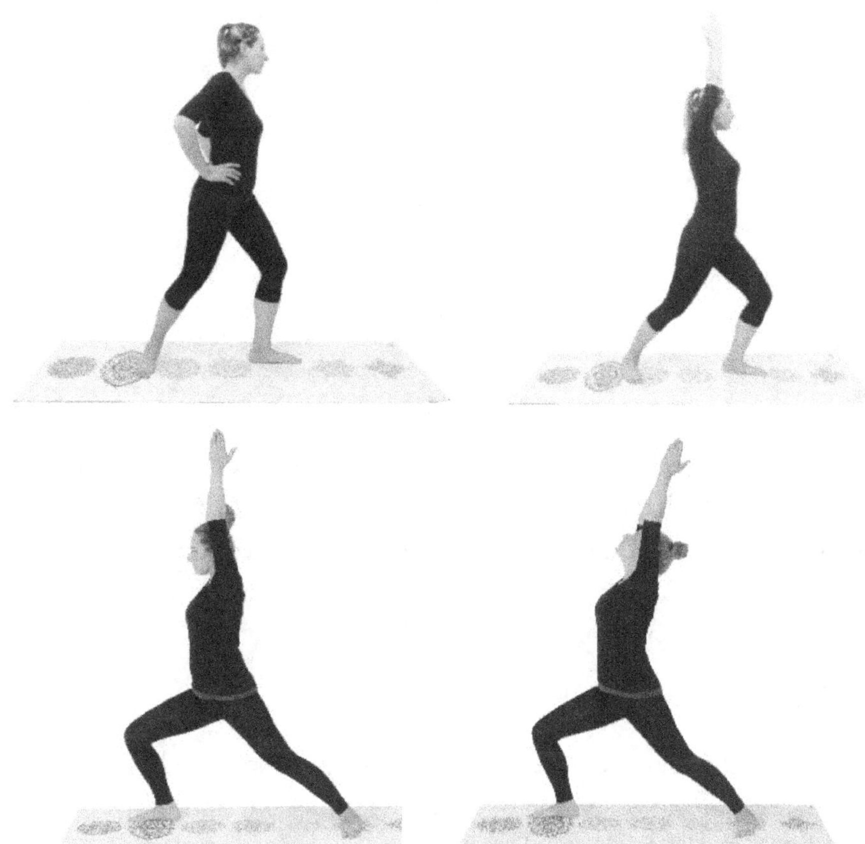

Practice: The leg positioning should be right foot opening on 90° degrees to the right side and the left foot should be on 45° degrees on diagonal position. Inhale to rest both hands on the waist with fingers facing forward. Exhale to bring the chest and upper body to the right side. Bend the right knee to your comfort and slightly push the hip forward. Some practitioners, and especially during the first and third trimester, are more comfortable on this position only. This is the starting position. Inhale to raise the hands up, where the inner upper arm is in same line to the ears. Continue breathing normally at the final pose. From second trimester onwards, can fix the gaze up to the raised hands, or if experiencing nausea, gaze to be fixed straight at the eye level. The hands can either be in Namaste Mudra or with the palms facing each other from a distance. Exhale to release the hands. Straighten the knee. From the chest return to the center.

Modification 1:

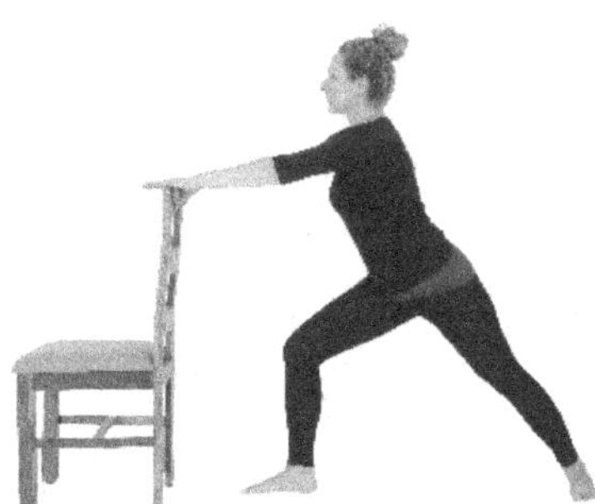

With the same leg positioning and starting position, can use the support of a chair to rest the hands on the back of the chair. The lower limb benefits can be the same, though the upper limb will have lowered stretching effects. With the support of a chair, practitioner can maintain the balance, especially from second trimester onwards.

Breathing: Normal breathing.

Awareness: Physical – on balancing the body while stretching the limbs and on synchronization of breath with the movement. Spiritual – on throat (vishuddhi) chakra, heart (anahata) chakra, solar plexus (manipura) chakra, sacral (swadhisthana) chakra or root (mooladhara) chakra.

Benefits: Strengthens the arm and leg muscles, shoulders and back region. Opens the chest and pelvis.

Precautions: Those with high blood pressure, heart conditions and hip, leg, knee injuries should avoid the practice.

Note: During the first trimester, the legs should be spread as much as it is the width of the yoga mat and the gaze should be fixed straight at the eye level to avoid dizziness.

From second trimester onwards legs can be wider apart, with the gaze fixed either straight at the eye level – if still experiencing dizziness, or fixed at the raised hands.

95. Warrior II – Virabhadrasana II

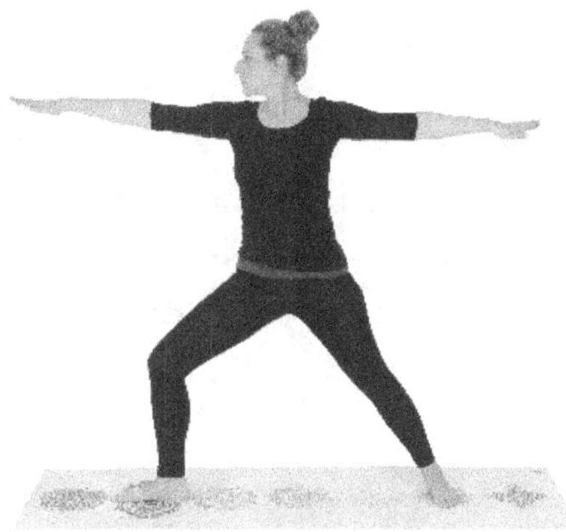

Practice: Similar positioning of the legs to Virabhadrasana I. Inhale to raise the arms open sideways to the shoulders' level. Bend the right leg pointing at 90° degrees. Turn the head looking to the right hand fingers and keep the chin parallel to the right arm. Breathe normally while in the position for 10-15 easy counts. Slowly straighten the knee, switch to the left side with the arms continuously open. Fix the left leg pointing at 90° degrees, look to the left hand fingers and the chin parallel to the left arm. Breathe normally while in the position for 10-15 easy counts. This is 1 round. Can practice 3-5 rounds.

Variation:

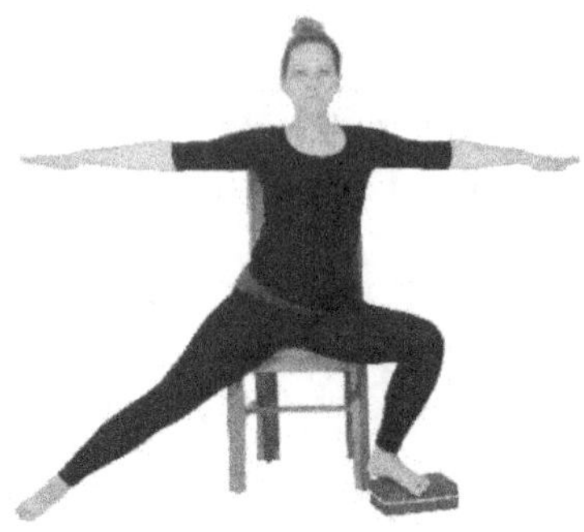

For those who experience severe nausea and especially during the third trimester when the practitioner has gained the pregnancy weight, to avoid knees' compression, can practice seated on a chair, though with lower effects. The legs and arms should be similarly positioned to the classic form of the practice. Can use the support of a yoga block to rest the foot on so the knee is bent (1 or 2 yoga blocks can be used, depending the chair size and the practitioner's height). Can be on the position for 10-15 easy counts with normal breathing. To release the position, exhale to bring the foot off the yoga block. Slide it the yoga block to the other side and repeat the same to complete 1 round. Can practice 3-5 rounds.

Variation: With the Baby

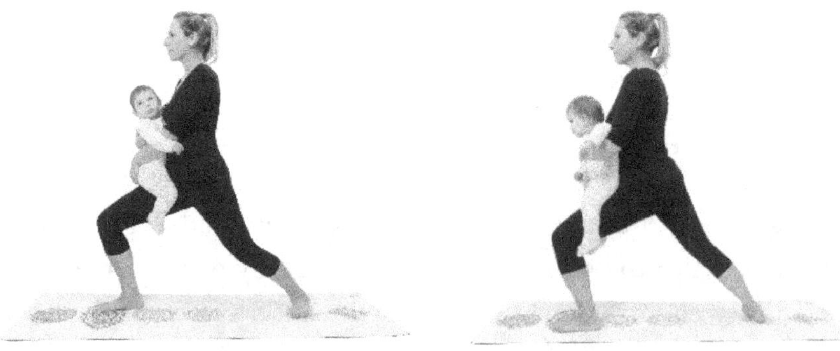

Choose the best baby positioning for you by holding the baby either facing you or with its back on you, and practice normally.

Breathing: Normal breathing on final position.

Awareness: Physical – on balancing the body while stretching the limbs and on synchronization of breath with the movement. Spiritual – on sacral (swadhisthana chakra) and root (mooladhara) chakra.

Benefits: Strengthens the arm and leg muscles, shoulders and back region. Opens the chest encouraging prana flow. Opens up the pelvis. Improves concentration and balance.

Precautions: Those with high blood pressure, heart conditions and hip, leg, knee injuries should avoid the practice.

Note: During the first trimester, the legs should be spread as much as it is the width of the yoga mat and the gaze should be fixed straight at the eye level to avoid dizziness. From second trimester onwards legs can be wider apart, with the gaze fixed either straight at the eye level – if still experiencing dizziness, or fixed at the hand on the same side of the bent knee. This practice is not needed to be practiced during third trimester, however, if practitioner insists, should only try the given variation.

96. Warrior III – Virabhadrasana III

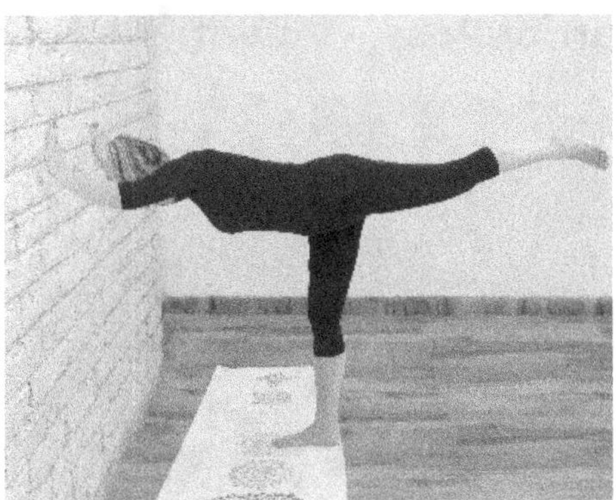

Practice: For this practice, the upper body is bent from the hip joint into 90° degrees. Should use the support of a wall to hold on with the palms of the hands against it to practice safely. Inhale to lift one leg up as much as 90° degrees high. Continue normal breathing for 10-15 easy counts. Exhale to bring down the lifted leg. Inhale to raise the other leg and repeat the same. This is 1 round and can repeat 3-5 rounds.

Modification 1: If feeling comfortable, can release hands one-by-one from the wall and with control bring them down under the shoulders' level. To maintain balance without strain can touch the fingers on the ground. Focus on having the spine aligned with the lower limb.

Modification 2: More experienced practitioners can bring the hands one-by-one behind and to the side of the buttocks with normal breathing. Focus on having the spine aligned with both limbs.

Breathing: Normal breathing on final position.

Awareness: Physical – retain the alignment of limbs and spine. Maintain the balance. Spiritual – on sacral (swadhisthana) or solar plexus (manipura) chakra.

Benefits: Strengthens the arms, back, hips and leg muscles. Helps on focus, concentration and nervous balance.

Precautions: Those with high blood pressure, heart and low back conditions should avoid this practice. Not to be practiced during third trimester.

97. Reverse Warrior Pose – Viparita Virabhadrasana

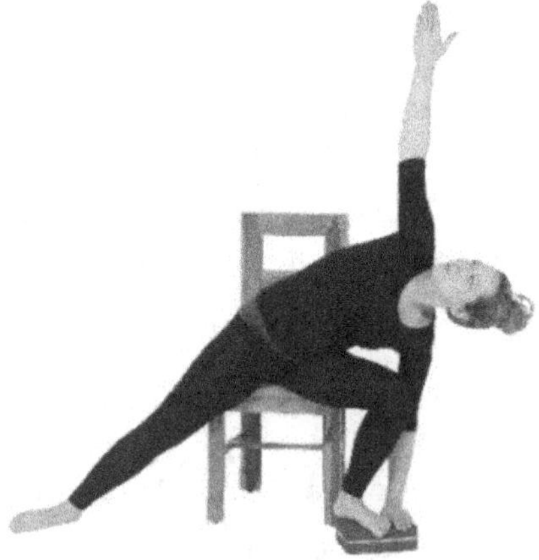

Practice: From Warrior II – Virabhadrasana II, seated on the chair variation, exhale to side bend to the left side with the right arm outstretched upwards and gaze at the fingers or look up straight. The left arm should be lowered to touch or hold on to the yoga block. Remain at this position for 2-3 comfortable breaths. On final position, breathe normally for 20 seconds. Inhale to bring T-shape arms to the center. Exhale to side bend to the right with the right hand sliding down the extended leg and the left hand stretched upwards by maintaining the T-shape, without any strain. Inhale to return to the center to complete 1 round. Can practice 3-5 rounds and repeat the same by changing the legs positioning.

Breathing: Inhale at the center and return to the center. Exhale to side bend. Normal breathing between the movements and at holding position.

Awareness: Physical – on synchronization of the breath with the movements and avoid over-bending/ overstretching. Spiritual – on sacral (swadhisthana) chakra or solar plexus (manipura) chakra.

Benefits: Stretches the sides of the torso and arms and helps open the hips.

Precautions: Those with shoulders, spinal, back, pelvic, hips, knees or ankle conditions should avoid this practice. Not to be practiced in complicated pregnancy.

Note: The seated variation can be performed from second trimester onwards. Every bending should happen from the waist and sideways with caution. There should be no abdomen engagement or jerky movements on the upper body. The extended leg and bending should feel comfortable.

Squatting Asanas

Squatting practices are only good for third trimester. During the first and fourth trimester there is no need for any squatting, as we aim to close the pelvic floor muscles and not open them up. In the second trimester there is no need for any squatting, especially until the first half, whereas from the second half you could maybe introduce half squatting practices such as modified Utkatasana and Kaliasana to start strengthening the body to welcome the full squats that is required to practice at the Third Trimester. All squatting practices are important on the third trimester, as these help the baby to come to correct position for birth.

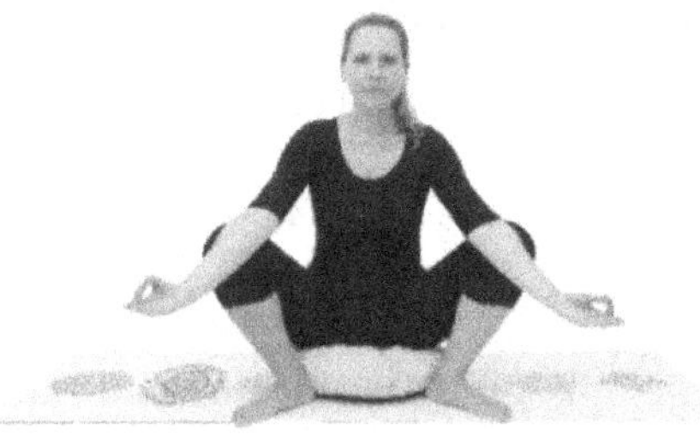

For some of the following asanas, it will be required to adopt the starting position of the modified Namaskarsana, by sitting on a cushion to avoid any pressure on the knees mostly.

98. Chair Pose – Utkatasana

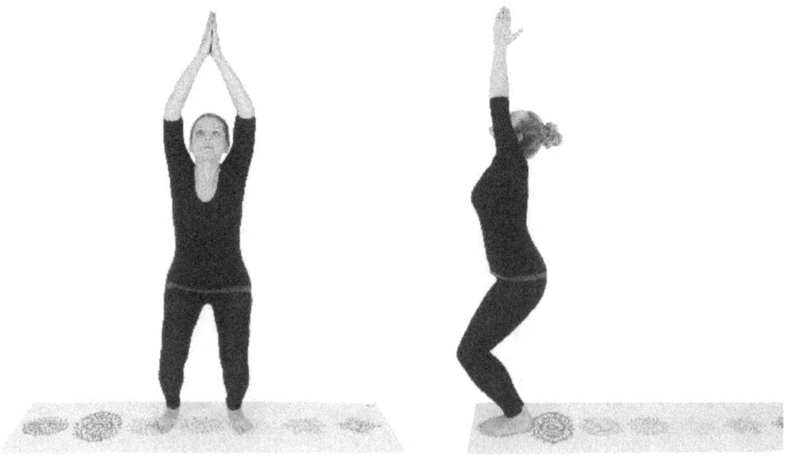

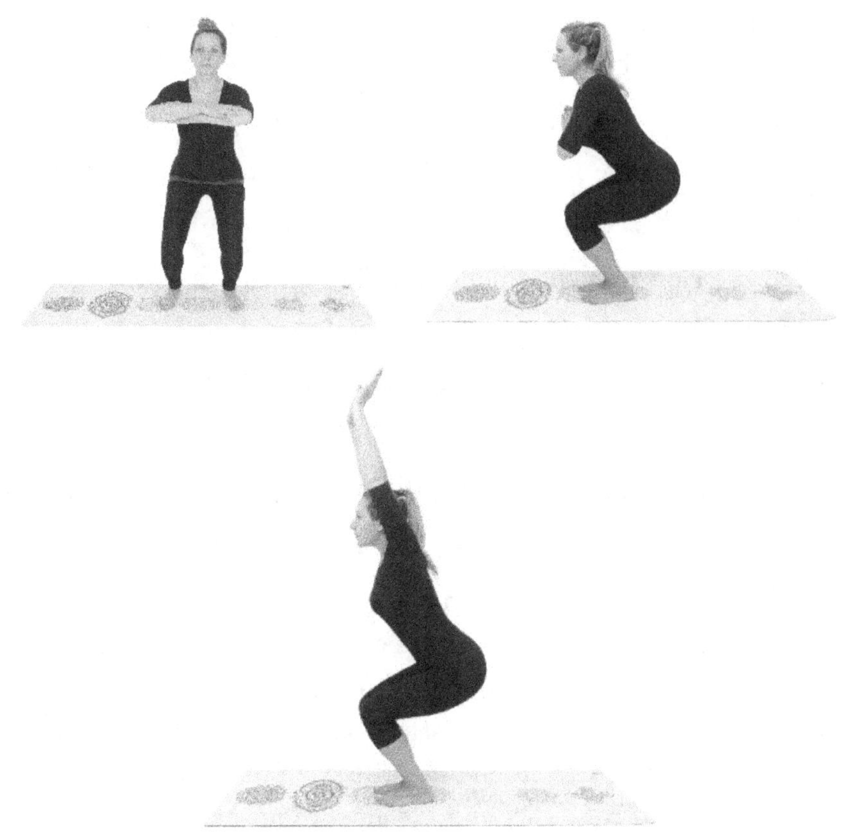

Practice: Standing in Tadasana, breathe deeply to relax the body completely. Stand erect with the feet open apart at approximately 1,5 feet ≈ 45 cm. The whole body weight should be on the heels, whereas the toes are light and not engaged.

Hands Modifications:

- Stretch the arms forward with palms facing downwards and elbows straight. Maintain them at this position throughout the practice.

- Stretch the arms forward with palms facing downwards and elbows straight. Inhale to bring them up with palms facing each other when bending the knees. Exhale to lower them in front of the body when returning to standing position.

- Stretch the hands to the side of the body and keep them there throughout the practice.

- Stretch the hands to the side of the body. Inhale to bring them up when bending the knees. Exhale to lower them when returning to standing position.

- Keep the hands on the thighs and slide up and down to the thighs with the movement.

- Interlock the arms in front of the chest where the left hand is holding the right elbow and the right hand is holding the left elbow.

- Keep the hands on Namaste Mudra in front of the chest when inhaling. On exhalation, bend the knees and raise the hands above the head.

Slowly inhale, lengthen the spine, and exhale to bend the knees by lowering the hips. Gently push the pelvis down as if sitting on a chair. Inhale to bring the body up and include the hands on the ideal positioning for the practitioner as above mentioned. Exhale to bring the hands and body down. Inhale to return to standing position. Can practice for 8-12 counts with continuous and controlled movement with no strain.

Variation 1:

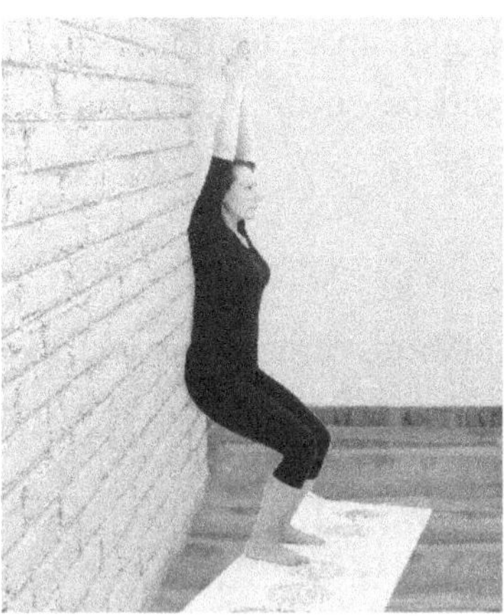

During the third trimester, can take the support of the wall to maintain balance. Create some gap between the heels and the wall [approximately

1 foot ≈ 30cm]; the space required depends on body capacity, and practitioner should adjust accordingly. Rest the buttocks and the upper back on the wall. The hands can either rest on the wall or the thighs or for experienced practitioners can be raised above the head when bending the knees and lowered when returning to standing position. The knees should bend forward with the knee caps looking to the front direction. Breathe deeply to relax the body completely. Inhale and exhale to bend the knees sliding down the wall from the lower and upper back. Inhale to straighten the knees and return to standing position. This is 1 count. Can practice for 8-12 counts with continuous and controlled movement with no strain. *OR* can remain static on final position for 1-2 minutes with normal breathing and the back always in contact with the wall.

Variation 2:

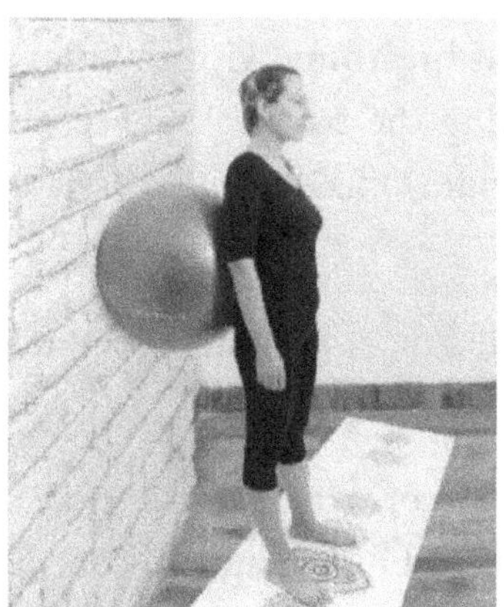
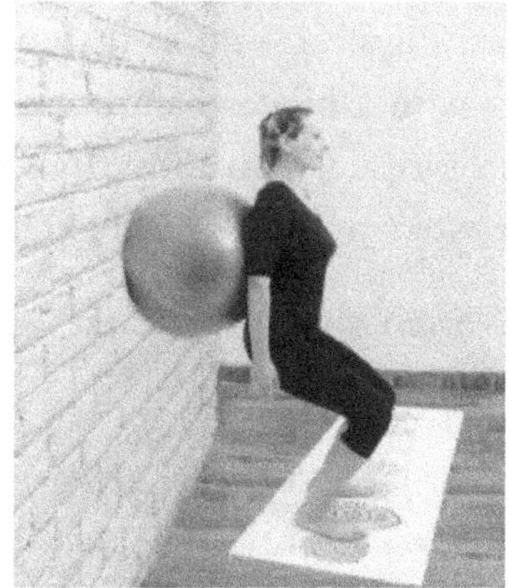

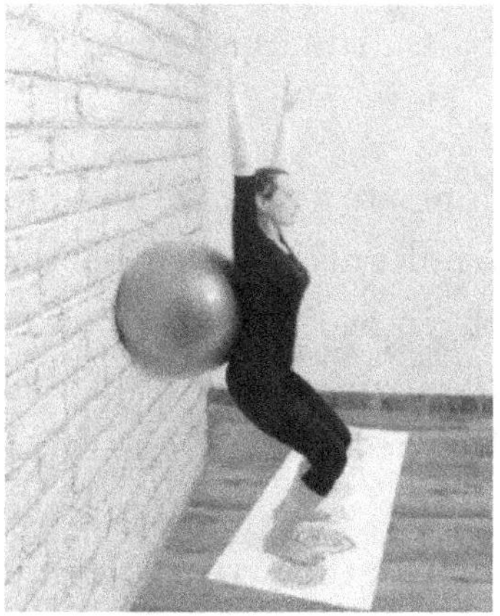

Similar to Variation 1. Use the support of a balancing pilates ball between the middle back and the wall. Adjust the ball to a comfortable position. Awareness must be sliding up and down with the ball always in contact with the wall. Movements must be controlled and smooth with no jerky effects on the body and the belly. The starting position should be leaning gently towards the wall with a squeeze effect on the ball to maintain its contact with the wall and the back. When bending the knees, the body goes down and should feel the ball around the shoulder blades. When returning to standing position, should feel the ball around the middle back area.

Breathing: Breathe normally to relax the body in starting position. Inhale to raise the hands up. Exhale to bent the knees. Inhale to return to standing position.

Awareness: Physical – on synchronized breathing with the movement; if practicing with a pilates ball, on keeping the balance between body, ball and wall. Spiritual – on throat (vishuddhi) chakra, sacral (swadhisthana) chakra or root (mooladhara) chakra.

Benefits: Strengthens the chest, spine, hips, thighs, knees and ankles muscles. Balances the body.

Precautions: Not to be practiced in case of chronic knee pain, arthritis, damaged ligaments, headache or insomnia. During the pre-conception and especially during menstruation should practice gently and with caution. Not recommended for first trimester practice and during the fourth trimester.

Note: This practice belongs to the squatting family and needs a lot of strength on the thighs and knees. When bending the knees, the knee caps must look forward. To avoid pressure on the knees, keep the feet wider open and move the body weight on the heels; otherwise, bending becomes more intense for the knees. Aim of this asana during pregnancy is not to keep the body alignment nor the small distance between the feet, but to massage and open the pelvic floor muscles. When practicing be aware of the lower back not to be arched on the way down. Instead, the tailbone should be tucked, and in the preconception and postnatal duration the core must be engaged. On second trimester can practice any of given variations with caution. On third trimester is advisable to use the support of a wall and/or balancing ball with the heels adjusted to a comfortable distance from the wall, to maintain a safe balance during the practice. If practitioner is comfortable, can practice any of the given variations during the third trimester. The distance of the feet apart, and the distance of the heels from the wall depends on individual practice, as every person has different body capacity, therefore, during the pregnancy the body must be adjusted to own comfort zone. It is not recommended to practice during the first trimester this or any squatting poses. Practitioners who are into yoga and practicing daily, some times more than once per day, should note that they should include this asana to their routine only once per day, either in the morning or on the evening.

99. Goddess Pose – Kaliasana

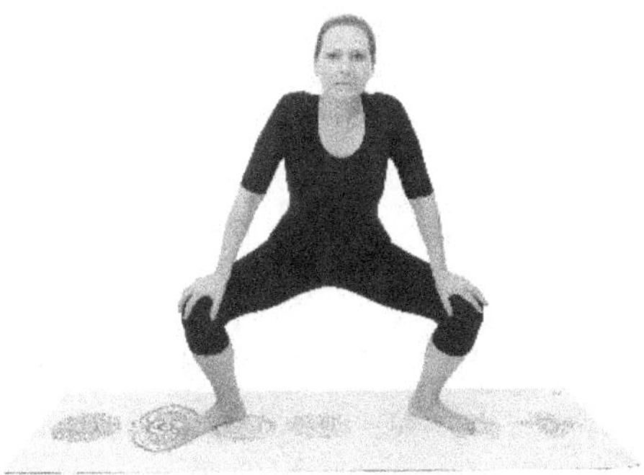

Practice: Standing in Samasthiti, breathe deeply to relax the body completely. Stand erect with the feet open apart at approximately 2-2,5 feet ≈ 60-75 cm gap. The legs should be diagonally open with the toes facing outwards. This is the starting position. Exhale to bend the knees to open diagonally to the side on a squatting position. Keep the hands on the thighs or knees, and allow natural sliding of the hands up and down to the thighs as the body comes up and down. Inhale to return to standing position. Can practice this 5-8 times as a warm up before introducing some of the other variations.

Variation 1:

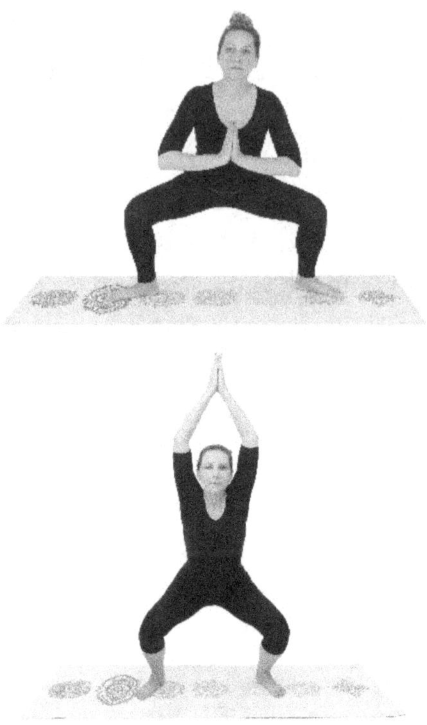

Inhale to bring the hands on Namaste Mudra in front of the chest and stay in that position for a few normal breaths. Inhale to lift the body up by keeping the knees bent to a certain level and raise the hands above the head. Exhale to a deeper squat and return the hands in front of the chest. Practice this for 5-8 times with continuous movement and controlled breathing.

Variation 2:

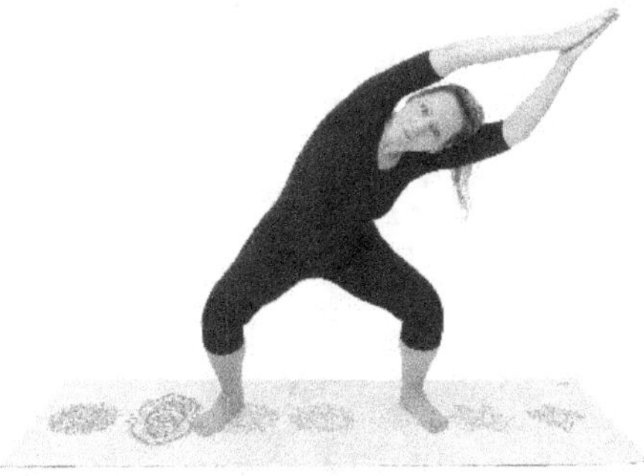

As in Variation 1, inhale to bring the hands on anjali mudra in front of the chest and stay in that position for a few normal breaths. Inhale to lift the body up by keeping the knees bent to a certain level and raise the hands above the head or keep them in front of the chest if it feels more comfortable. Exhale to bend upper body sideways. Inhale to the center.

Exhale to the other side. Inhale to the center. This is 1 count. Can practice 5-8 counts with continuous movement and controlled breathing.

Variation 3:

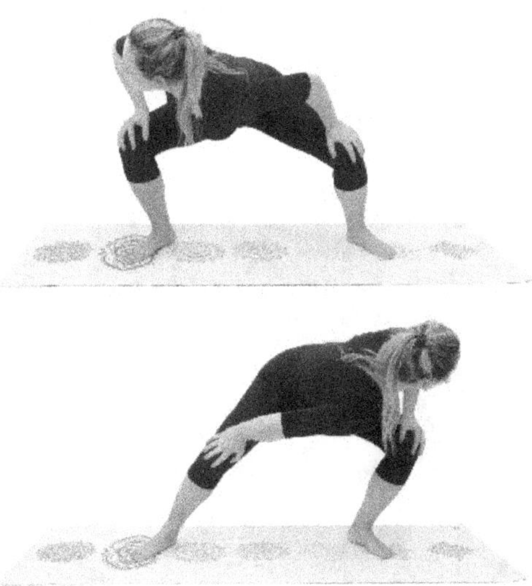

From starting position, exhale to bend the knees to open diagonally to the side on a squatting position. Keep the hands on the thighs or knees, and allow natural movement of the hands as the body twists gently from side to side, like a dancing move. The movement should be happening from the knees. Inhale to twist to the right, exhale to the center, inhale to twist to the left, exhale to the center. This is 1 count. Can practice this 5-8 counts with continuous movement and controlled breathing.

Modification:

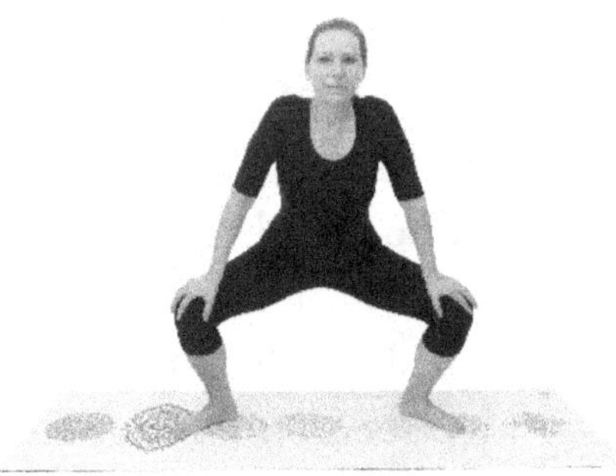

If practitioner finds it challenging to balance with the twist move, can keep the trunk in natural position and slightly move like a dance move from right to left continuously with steady movement and normal breathing. The heels should always be in firm contact with the ground allowing a rhythmic move with the toes relaxed. This practice gives a nice massage to the pelvic floor muscles. Can practice this 5-8 counts with continuous movement and normal breathing. Exhale to slowly come back to standing position.

Variation 4:

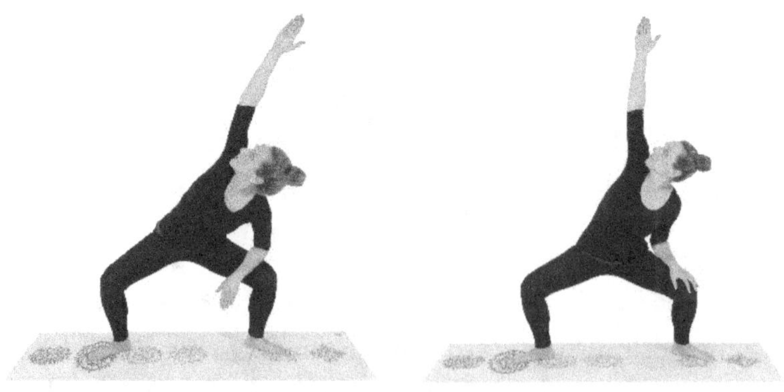

From starting position, exhale to bend the knees to open diagonally to the side on a squatting position. Place the right elbow on the right thigh just above the knee; or the hand on the knee. Inhale to raise the left arm up, extend it upwards and gaze at the extended hand, or look straight. Follow the body on the move. If placing the elbow on the thigh, the body automatically will come lower to the side and will give a bigger stretch feeling on the sides. If the hand is placed on the knee, the body curves less, however the stretch is equally effective.

Variation 5:

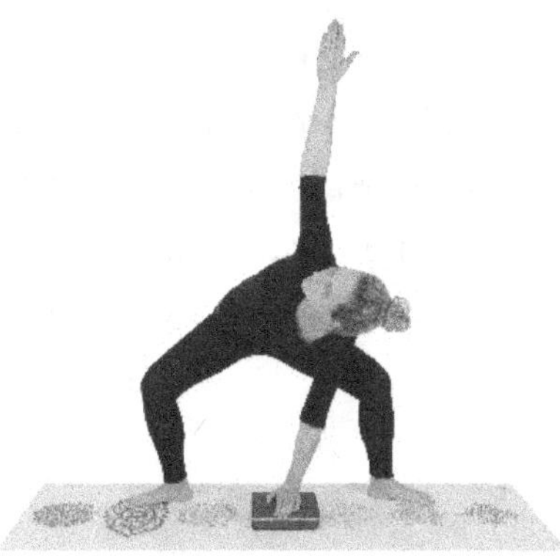

For a deeper squat and greater stretch, can use the support of a yoga block. Keep the yoga block in the center of the body, just in front of you and place one hand on top of it. Yoga Block can be vertical or horizontal, according the level of depth practitioner feels comfortable to practice. Inhale to raise the left arm up, extend it upwards and gaze at the extended hand, or look straight. Stay in that position for 2-3 normal breaths. Repeat the same with the other hand to complete 1 round. Can practice 5-8 rounds.

Variation 6:

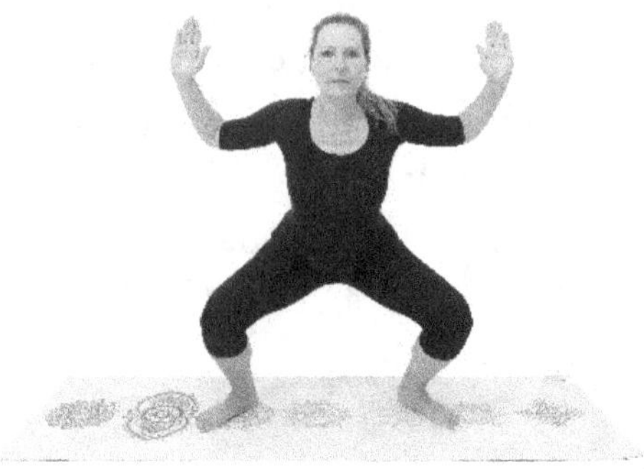

From starting position, exhale to bend the knees to open diagonally to the side on a squatting position. Inhale to open the hands to the side for chest opening. Stay for 2-3 normal breaths in that position. Exhale to come up to standing position by releasing the hands. This is 1 count. Can practice 5-8 counts. Advanced practitioners can try this asana on their toes and maybe with a wall support.

Variation 7:

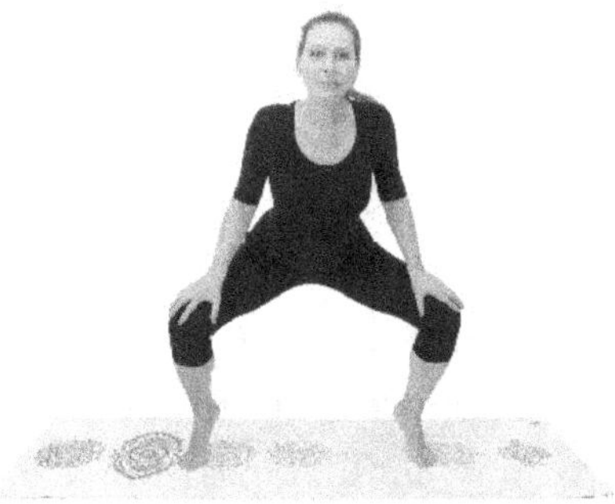

In all variations, after childbirth and when the body has fully recovered from labor, can come on balancing on the toes up and down with synchronized breath-movement or continuous breathing with rapid movements up and down. The heels should not touch the ground on the downward movement. This practice will benefit core engagement and strength as well as strengthening the whole back side of the lower limbs, particularly the cuff muscles. Can practice this 8-10 times with slow movement up and down as 1 set, and 8-10 times with rapid movement. Gradually, and the strength is building up, practitioner can increase repetitions to 10-15 and 15-20.

Variation: With the Baby

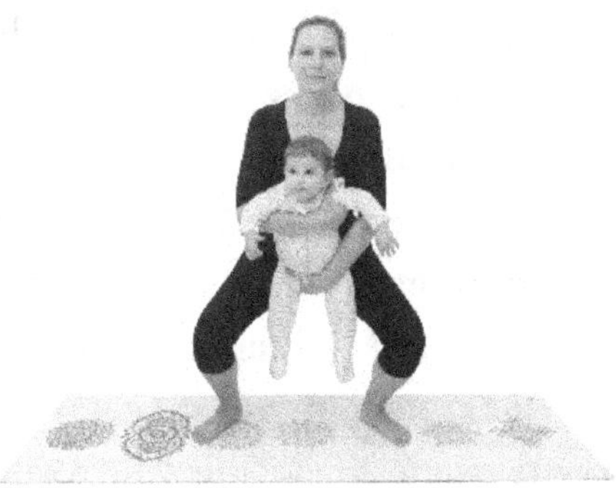

Similarly, grasp the baby to safety and practice the feet variation(s) you feel more comfortable with.

Breathing: Normal breathing with continuous movement.

Awareness: Physical – with the hands movement on shoulders, chest and rib cage; with the squatting on engaging the calves, hamstrings, hips and pelvic floor and on breathing. Spiritual – on root (mooladhara) chakra or sacral (swadhisthana) chakra.

Benefits: While squatting, the asana works as a hip opener, massages the pelvic floor muscles and stretches the gluteal muscles. Stimulates the uro-genital system and pelvic floor. Opens, stretches and strengthens the shoulder joints, the chest, and the whole lower limb and all its muscles. With the dynamic practicing, the blood gets circulated better, the nerves and the muscles are getting activated.

Precautions: For those suffering from arthritis, it is recommended to practice the knee movements from Pawanmuktasana Series, and not Kaliasana or any other squatting pose, because of the intense pressure on the lower limb joints. In such cases, practitioner should be actually seated on a chair with way less benefits from the practice.

Note: To avoid pressure on the knees, keep the knees wider open so the genital area is also wider open during the squatting position. Also, body weight should be on the heels to release pressure from the knees; otherwise, bending becomes more intense for the knees. Aim of this asana during pregnancy is not to keep the alignment of knees and ankles, because there should be no holding on the squatting position. The movement has to be continuous and the knees take less pressure that way. Intention is to massage and open the pelvic floor muscles. It is not recommended to practice during the first trimester this or any squatting poses. This asana is highly recommended during the third trimester and its practice has to be more dynamic instead of static, because we need the would-be-mum's body to be active. With the extra body weight and the size of the belly that changes the body gravity, static practicing will require core engagement which is not recommended at any phase of a pregnancy; it may also create a cramp to the inner thighs area. Therefore, movement has to be continuous and dynamic. Experienced practitioners with yogic background can easily preform Kaliasana with no restrictions. The moment the legs start shivering, the cuff muscles burning, the hamstrings are shaking, the practice must stop at once and go to a relaxed position. Practitioners who are into yoga and practicing daily, some times more than once per day, should note that they should include this asana to their routine only once per day, either in the morning or on the evening.

100. Twist and Chest Opening Pose

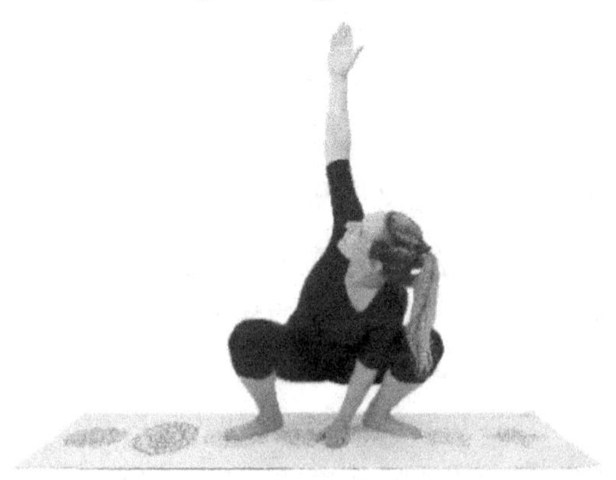

Practice: Start from the modified Namaskarsana while seated on a cushion. Position the palms of the hands in front of the body and between the knees. Inhale, open the chest and take the right hand up. Exhale to lower it back to the ground. Inhale to raise the left hand up. Exhale to lower it back to the ground. This is 1 round. Can practice 10-12 rounds.

Breathing: Normal breathing on starting position. Inhale to raise the hand up. Exhale to lower it back to the ground.

Awareness: Physical – on breath synchronization with the movement and on not compressing or hitting the belly. Spiritual – on sacral (swadhisthana) chakra and root (mooladhara) chakra.

Benefits: Elevates back pain. Opens up the chest and helps respiratory system. Stretches the pelvic floor muscles.

Precautions: Those with ankle, knee, wrist, shoulder, back or spinal injuries should avoid the practice.

101. Squatting Toe Balance Pose – Jangha Shakti Vikasaka

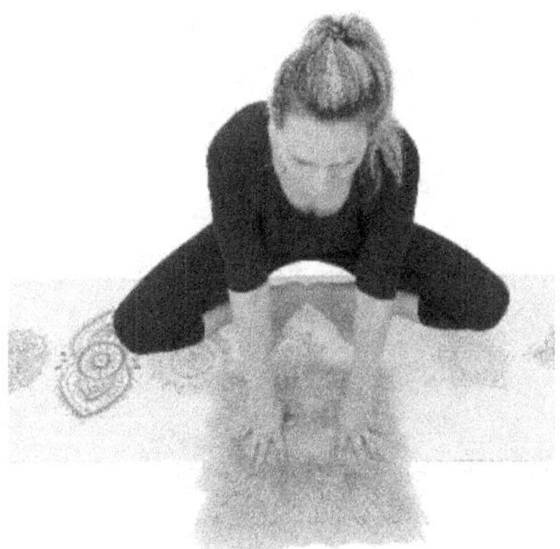

Practice: Start from Namaskarsana, with the knees wide apart, balance on the toes and bring the heels together. Non experienced practitioners can use the support of a cushion or yoga block to hold onto to come to position. Stay in the position for 2-3 comfortable breaths. When ready, inhale to lean to one side by bringing one knee closer to the floor, in a circular movement. Exhale to lean to the other side with continuous movement and breathing. This is 1 round. Can practice 3-5 rounds or more for experienced practitioners.

Modification:

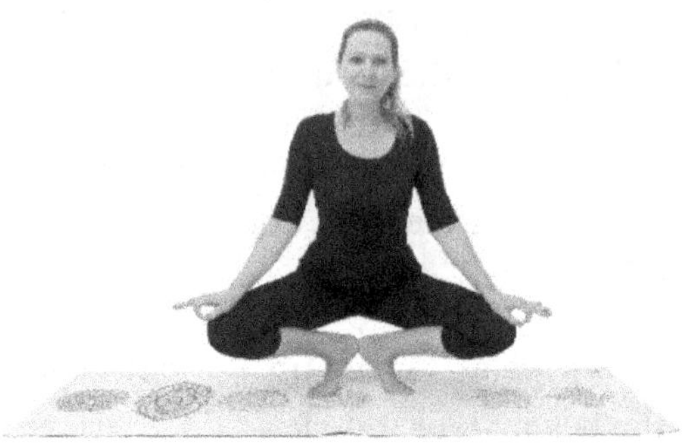

From Namaskarsana, with the knees wide apart, balance on the toes and bring the heels together. Position the palms face down on the knees – can adopt Jnana Mudra, or for better balance can open the arms sideways. Stay in the position for 2-3 comfortable breaths. When ready, inhale to lean to one side by bringing one knee closer to the floor. Exhale to lean to the other side with continuous movement and breathing. This is 1 round. Can practice 3-5 rounds or more for experienced practitioners.

Breathing: Normal breathing.

Awareness: Physical – on breathing and balancing with the movement and on not compressing or hitting the belly. Spiritual – on sacral (swadhisthana) chakra and root (mooladhara) chakra.

Benefits: Stretches and strengthens the pelvic floor muscles and inner thighs. Shapes the thighs. Massages the perineum.

Precautions: Those suffering from sciatica, or with ankle, knee, hips or back conditions should avoid the practice.

Practice-Note: This practice may be challenging for beginner level practitioners. Can attempt practice with the support of a wall.

102. Duck Walking – Karandavasana

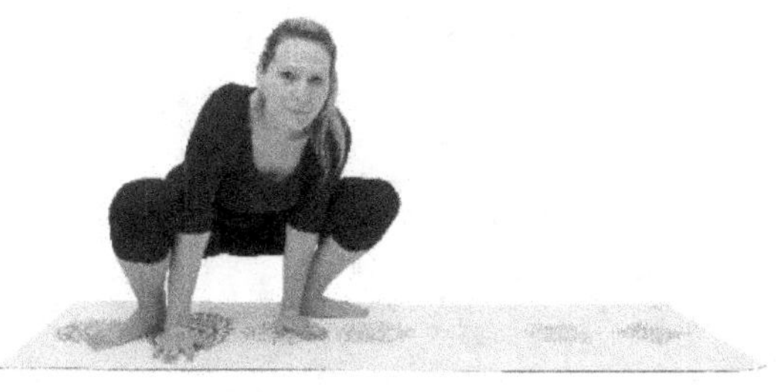

Practice: From Namaskarsana, slowly place the palms of the hands on the ground in front of the body and come on the toes. Gently and slowly step one foot out to the side and walk the hands forward. Take the other foot out and keep walking with the hands one step, following by one leg at a time. Can practice as many steps it feels comfortable to.

Breathing: Normal breathing.

Awareness: Physical – on stepping and opening the foot to the side to avoid belly compression or be hit. Spiritual – on sacral (swadhisthana) chakra and root (mooladhara) chakra.

Benefits: Increases flexibility in the pelvic floor muscles. Tones the whole lower limb. Stretches and strengthens the back.

Precautions: Should not be practiced by people with high blood pressure, arteriosclerosis, ankle or knee problems and sciatica.

Note: Only advanced practitioners should practice this asana on their third trimester only. Those who are using squat toilets, or would-be-mums who are used to mop the floor by hand and cloth, may find it easier to practice. Otherwise, during pregnancy should practice only on third trimester and only if practice is done with comfort.

103. Bridge or Shoulder Pose – Kandharasana or Setu Bandha Sarvangasana

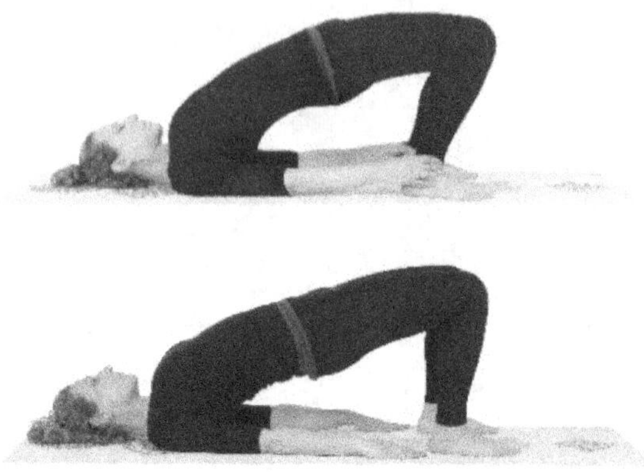

Practice: During pre-conception, first and towards the end of fourth trimester, come to Shavasana and bend the knees with the soles flat on the ground and the heels touching the buttocks. Keep the knees and feet at hip width apart. Can hold the ankles with the hands, or keep the hands flat and straight to the side and parallel to the body. This is the starting position. Inhale to raise from the hips and arch the back upwards, raise the chest up to the chin and navel to maximum body capacity without any strain. The shoulders and feet should remain still during the practice. Hold the position for 3-5 counts and slowly lower the body to starting position on exhalation. To release the pose, release the hands from the ankles, slowly move further away the heels from the body and outstretch legs to relax. Practice 5-10 rounds and release hands from the ankles before outstretching the legs.

Variation 1:

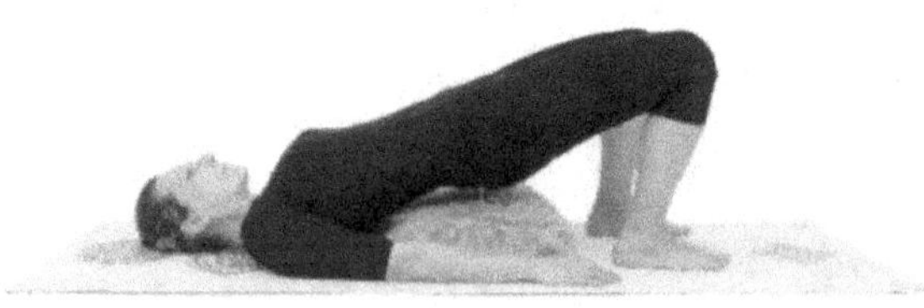

Sit in Sukhasana and place a cushion on the lower back to lie down on it. Lie on the floor from the side with the support of the hands. Bend the knees with the soles flat on the ground. Adjust the position so that lumbar is on the cushion, the feet are comfortably positioned as wide apart (minimum 1.5 feet ≈ 45cm) and as close to the buttocks; in any case, position must feel comfortable. With a mild move from the hips, inhale to raise the body upwards. Exhale to lower the body. To release the pose, slowly move further away the heels from the body and outstretch legs to relax. During the second and third trimester, can stay in the upward position for 1 breath, or can practice in slow and continuous movements up and down. Practice 5-10 rounds

Breathing: Normal breathing to come to position. Inhale to lift body up. Exhale to lower the body.

Awareness: Physical – on the movement from the hips and breathing. Spiritual – on throat (vishuddhi) chakra or heart (anahata) chakra

Benefits: In the pre-conception time, it tones the female reproductive organs and helps on menstrual disorders. It can prevent miscarriage. Strengthens and helps realign the spine, opens the chest area, eliminates rounded shoulders. Strengthens and tones the pelvic floor muscles, hips, abdomen and lumbar. Can relieve backache. Stretches the abdominal organs and colon, improving digestive system and help on constipation. In late pregnancy, helps a breech baby to come into position.

Precautions: Those suffering from digestive disorders such as acidity and heartburns, or abdominal hernia should not practice this asana.

Note: Many women are not able to move the belly up and many are mistaking the practice by engaging the core. The support of a cushion between the lumbar and the ground is necessary for two reasons: a) the back should not be flat on the ground especially during late pregnancy, because it has the same effects of any supine pose with inferior vena cava compression; and b) many women cannot move easily during their late pregnancy, and while in any supine position the body should be little higher than the floor to allow less effort for the movements. With the grown belly, the chest should not to be lifted with the upward movement, because automatically there is a stretch on the skin between the chest, thorax and upper abdomen area. Overstretching when lifting higher the body, will create excess pressure on the lumbar area and should never allow practitioner to go higher than 15cm during this practice. With the chest not lifted up, practitioner can maintain better balance and stillness while practicing. Should perform before or after a forward bend.

Pranayama is defined as breath control or breath work and can be beneficial, whether a practitioner is ready to conceive, is already carrying, or recovering from childbirth.

Prana, the *Life Force* or *Vital Energy*, is more about the air or oxygen we breathe into our lungs, whereas,

Ayama is the Control, the Expansion or Extension of the prana dimension.

The pranayama techniques can help activate and regulate the life force so the practitioner can expand own breathing capacity and by that way can increase awareness and vibratory energy. When one is ready to conceive or is already carrying, should totally avoid any breath holding or heating practices, such as:

- Agnisara Kriya (Activating the Digestive Fire)

- Bhastrika Pranayama (Bellows Breath)

- Kapalbhati and Kapalbhati Pranayama (Frontal Brain Cleansing)

- Uddiyana Bandha (Abdominal Contraction)

In the pre and postnatal period, women love learning breathing and pranayama techniques. It is beneficial for a woman to simply place her awareness on the feeling of her breath, as this will naturally slow and deepen the breath. The slow and deep breathing naturally calms the nervous system, helps feeling relaxed, connect with her baby in the prenatal period and to her inner self at all times. Most yoga teachers only teach 1, 2 or 3 pranayama techniques, which is a real shame for their students! Prana is the gift of life, and by giving this gift to a student can be truly a life changing experience, which many may develop as a good and healthy habit throughout their entire life.

The following pranayama techniques are safe, simple and effective breathing techniques which can be practiced by any wishing-to-be or would-be-mum. In the postnatal period, all pranayama techniques can be practiced. Particularly from second trimester onwards, a connection between mother and baby can be set in many ways and levels. During the class opening or closing when is mostly common to practice the pranayama techniques, as well as during practicing and resting, the connection can be established by gently touching the belly or even by mentally transferring prana to the baby.

Time of practice: All pranayama techniques and mudras is best practiced early in the morning or late in the evening, as during these times there is usually maximum quiet.

Starting position: Sit on a comfortable position from the Meditation Asanas on the mat or on a chair. The head and spine should be aligned and upright, the body relaxed and the eyes closed.

104. Yogic Breathing

The whole process of yogic breathing is a smooth, harmonious, natural breathing flow, where the body should be relaxed without any strain nor jerks.

Take a few breaths to normalize breathing. With the whole body relaxed, when ready, take a deep and slow inhalation where the abdomen fully expands and have the sensation the lungs are filling up with air. At the end of inhalation where the abdomen is expanded, start expanding the chest to feel the expansion outward and upward. The sensation should be fully expanding the rib cage, at which point inhale a little more to sense more air filling the upper lobes of the lungs. During this inhalation process, the shoulders and collar bone slightly move up following the breathing pattern in upper body expansion, which may give a tension in the neck muscles. This is one inhalation.

Continue to exhalation without any holding, by first relaxing the lower neck and upper chest, following the chest contraction downward and inward. Push the diaphragm towards the chest and feel the abdomen gently and smoothly without any force contracting towards the spine in an attempt to empty the lungs10[11]. This is one exhalation and completes 1 round.

To come back from the breathing practice, relax and start coming back to normal breathing by observing the breath. Slowly bring the awareness back to the physical body and the surroundings before opening the eyes.

Duration: Practice 5-10 rounds or more if needed.

Benefits: Yogic breathing helps practitioner to connect with own breath and correct poor breathing habits as well as increase oxygen intake. The full breath strengthens and engages the lungs, and calms the nervous system. With every inhalation the expansive breath carries more oxygen to the lungs and bloodstream, which in turn will improve body cells' oxygenation and circulation. With every exhalation, toxins and pollution trapped in the lower lobes of the lungs are released. Mentally, with each exhalation can also release worries, anxiety, anger, pain and any negative thought. With each breath, feel the cleansing and purifying effect and the stress levels reduce, and enjoy the relaxation effect connecting body and mind. Can be practiced softly during yoga nidra, meditation or relaxation.

Precautions: Should not be performed repetitively as an only pranayama technique. Should start with yogic breathing and add at least 1 or 2 more techniques during pranayama practicing.

---

[11] Normally, practitioner should push the diaphragm towards the chest and feel the abdomen contracting towards the spine trying to empty the lungs.

105. Anulom Vilom – Nadi Shodhana Pranayama

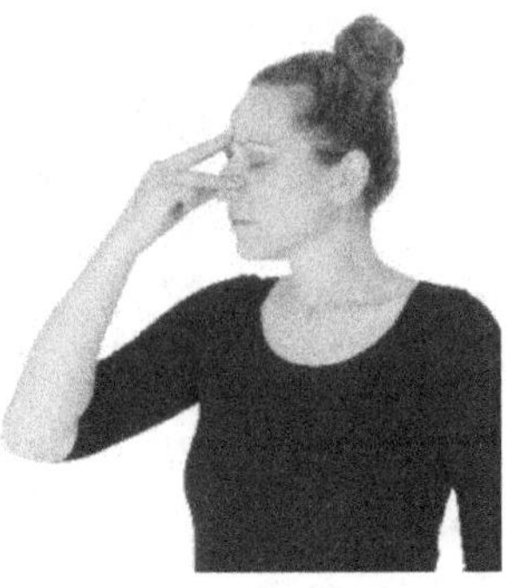

This practice is commonly known as Alternate Nostril Breathing, which alternate nostril breathing is only one of the many techniques of practicing anulom vilom. Out of the different techniques of anulom vilom, during pregnancy only the following two variations are recommended for safe practicing.

Practice: Practice Yogic Breathing for a few breaths to find breath awareness. The left hand should be rested on the left knee or can adopt Jnana Mudra. The right hand should be on Nosetip Position – Nasagra Mudra to start the practice.

Variation 1: Single Nostril Breathing

Close the right nostril with the thumb and breathe normally (inhale/ exhale) using only the left nostril for 5 times. Upon completion of the 5 breaths, release the thumb from the right nostril and close the left nostril with the ring finger. Breathe normally (inhale/ exhale) using only the right nostril for 5 times. Breathing rate should be normal. Lower the hands and breathe normally for 5 times through both nostrils to complete 1 round. Can practice 5-10 rounds.

Variation 2: Alternate Nostril Breathing

Close the right nostril with the thumb and inhale from the left nostril. On inhalation, mentally count 3 times "Om". Simultaneously, close the left nostril with the ring finger and release the thumb from the right one and on exhalation mentally count 3 times "Om". The "Om" counting during inhalation and exhalation keeps the time equal. Repeat the same with both nostrils to complete 1 round. Can practice 5-10 rounds.

Awareness: Physical – on synchronization of fingers movement with breathing. Spiritual – on third eye (ajna) chakra.

Benefits: Its practice calms the nervous system and balances both brain hemispheres, since both nostrils are separately used and brain cells get oxygenated. More air from the left nostril cherishes the analytical part of the brain and activates the ida nadi or chandra (moon) nadi which is for cool. When more air is inhaled by the right nostril, the creative part of the brain gets cherished and activates the pingala nadi or surya (sun) nadi, which is for heat. Strengthens and expands the lung capacity and brings a refreshing effect to the practitioner, if practiced frequently. With this exercise, the nervous system calms and eases stress and anxiety; and the breath comes back to balance, which in turn will improve physical, mental and emotional well-being. When feeling disconnected can help reconnect, focus and concentrate.

Precautions: People with high blood pressure, cardiac related issues, during pregnancy, or during the postnatal period, if the woman is suffering from postpartum depression breathing should be normal and continuous without holding. It should not be practiced during a cold, flu or fever.

106. Ocean or Psychic Breath – Ujjayi Pranayama

Would-be-mum can place one hand on the heart or chest area and the other on the belly. Inhale/ exhale for a few breaths through the nostrils by bringing the awareness on the nostrils. Inhale/ exhale for a few more long, deep and controlled breaths with the awareness brought to the throat and mentally feel the breath traveling through the throat. As the breathing becomes smoother, on exhalation gently contract the glottis in an attempt to have a soft and quiet snoring sound produced in the throat, audible only to the practitioner. The sound could also be a light 'Haaa' for beginner practitioners or those having difficulty to contract the glottis.

Duration: Can practice 10-15 breaths.

Precautions: Should not be practiced by those who experience agoraphobia or are introverted by nature, as well as those who have cold and cough symptoms. Practitioners suffering from slipped disc spinal cord conditions can practice in Vajrasana. If at any time during practice the would-be-mum feels lightheaded or heated up should stop the breathing practice.

Note: When practicing Ujjayi Pranayama, we constrict the throat muscles to create the sound, which should not feel forced or strong. Both inhalation and exhalation should be felt light, quiet, effortless and smooth. The awareness should be placed on the inner world – physical body and mind, calm the breath, calm the face muscles. It is a safe practice during pregnancy, as long as it is practiced softly, otherwise may have an inner heating effect. Generally, Ujjayi Pranayama helps practitioner to connect to the sound of own breath and inner self by creating a rhythm which improves focus, concentration and grounds in a meditative state of mind. It is beneficial to be practiced during pregnancy, as it softens the focus on body intensity which is perfect for labor and childbirth. Can be practiced softly during yoga nidra, meditation or relaxation.

107. Shhh Breath

With the eyes closed, place one hand on the heart or chest area and the other hand on the belly. Inhale deeply through the nostrils and exhale through the mouth by making a 'Shhh' sound. This is 1 round and can repeat 5-10 times.

Note: Similar to Ujjayi Pranayama, this breathing practice is very calming while the awareness is placed on the 'Shhh' sound. Both inhalation and exhalation should be felt light, quiet, effortless and smooth. It is a safe practice during pregnancy, as long as it is practiced softly, otherwise may have an inner heating effect. It is beneficial to be practiced during pregnancy, as it will naturally lengthen the breath which is perfect for labor and childbirth, and can also help feel calm.

If at any time during practice the mother-to-be feels lightheaded or heated up should stop the breathing practice.

108. Humming Bee Breath – Bhramari Pranayama

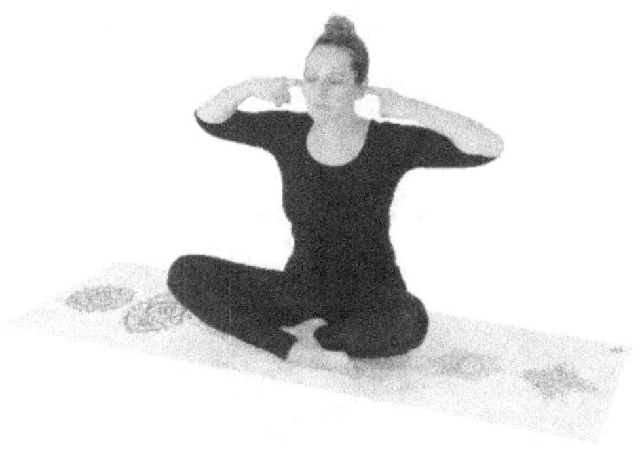

Bhramari means "bee" and its practice arises from the humming sound the bee makes. The sound is the Makkar sound from the sounds generated when chanting "Hum".

Practice: With the eyes closed, relax the whole body. Bring the hands to the ears and use the index or middle finger to close or plug the ears. The hands should be parallel to the ground. Keep the lips gently closed with the teeth slightly separated during the practice to allow the sound vibration of "Hum" to be heard and felt clearly within the head. During practicing, awareness should be brought to the heart (ajna) chakra and the body should remain motionless. Take a deep inhale through the nostrils and a slow controlled long exhale with the humming sound. At the end of exhalation, continue to the next round by maintaining the hand positioning; or can bring the hands down to the knees to Jnana Mudra to complete 1 round.

Duration: Normally 5-10 rounds. Practitioners with mental tension or anxiety can slowly increase to 10-15 minutes and up to 30 minutes.

Awareness: Physical – on breathing and on the humming sound within the head. Spiritual – on heart (ajna) chakra.

Benefits: It stimulates the pituitary gland and relaxes the nervous system. Feelings such as irritation, frustration, anxiety, anger, short temper can be benefited by this practice. Promotes focus, awareness and concentration. Beneficial for women suffering from postpartum depression.

Precautions: Not to be practiced by those who suffer from ear infections. Practice should not be performed on a supine position, but only on a seated and comfortable pose.

109. Closing the Seven Gates – Shanmukhi Mudra

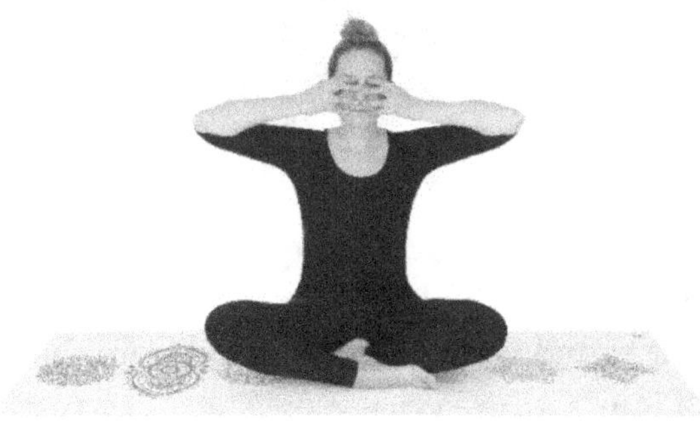

Although Shanmukhi Mudra is not a pranayama technique, it can be easily incorporated to Yogic Breathing. With this practice we symbolically shut all the senses using both our hands.

Practice: Raise the elbows and keep them parallel to the ground – this sitting position helps on focusing on the breathing. Close the eyes using the thumbs; the index fingers are gently placed on the eyelashes; the middle fingers are placed on top of the nostrils; the ring fingers are placed just below the nostrils and above the lips; the little fingers are placed at the brow of the lips.

Gently release the middle fingers from the nostrils to inhale slowly and deeply, using the yogic breathing. When inhalation is complete, close the nostrils again with the middle fingers and hold the breath for as long as it feels comfortable, and release again the middle fingers from the nostrils to slowly exhale. This action completes 1 round. Immediately continue to the next round. At the end of the practice, with the eyes closed, lower the hands to the knees and slowly bring awareness to the external sounds and the physical body.

Duration: Can practice 5-10 times or up to 30 minutes for experienced practitioners.

Awareness: Physical – on synchronizing the middle fingers press/release movement with the breath. Spiritual – on back of the head (bindu), third eye (ajna), or heart (anahata) to increase concentration. Aim of this practice is to withdraw from the senses.

Benefits: In the physical level, hands' and fingers' heat and energy relax the facial nerves and muscles. In the mental level, the mind gets quiet. In the spiritual level, enhances withdrawal from the senses. Shutting off the senses ensures that the sensation of senses don't reach the respective nerve centers in the brain, which in turn help the mind to be more focused and concentrated.

Precautions: Women suffering from postpartum depression should not practice.

Note: During the practice, one could hear many subtle sounds in the region of bindu chakra11F[12] or none at all. This comes with experience and practice. If hearing a sound, place the awareness to that sound. As sensitivity advances, and sounds are heard, the bindu chakra starts opening up and glowing its benefits to the body, mind and soul.

---

[12] Bindu chakra is located at the top back of the skull and is connected to the pineal gland. It is called the Moon Centre or The source of Ambrosia.

Mudra

1. **Prayer Hands or Namaste Mudra – Anjali Mudra**

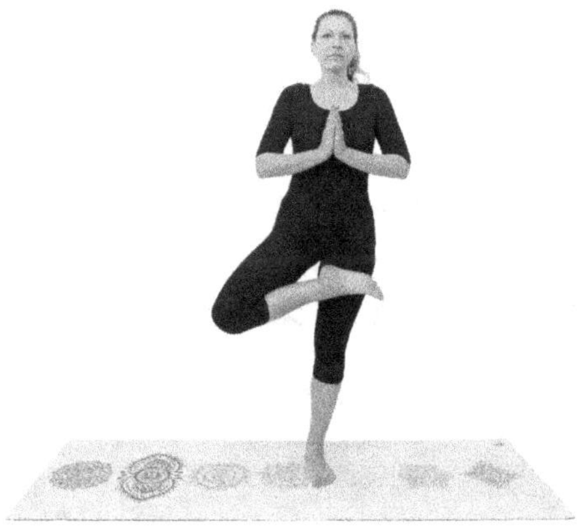

With the palms of the hands in contact and close to the chest, one can salute and greet others in daily life, promoting respect for oneself and others; and while practicing yoga can enhance concentration and balance.

2. **Nosetip Position – Nasagra Mudra**

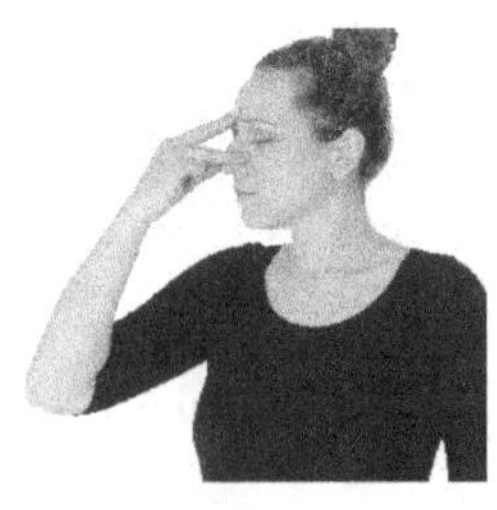

Bring the fingers of the right hand in front of the face, touch the eyebrow center with the index and middle fingers. The thumb is above the right nostril and the ring finger above the left nostril. The little finger is comfortably folded.

3. **Psychic Gesture of Knowledge – Jnana Mudra**

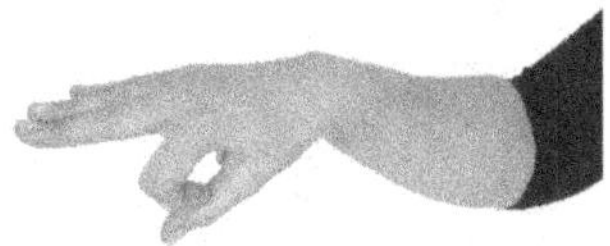

To practice, fold the index finger to touch the inner root of the thumb. The other three fingers should be straightened but relaxed and slightly apart. Relax the arms and bring the hand on the knee with the palm facing downward.

4. **Attitude of the Womb or Source – Yoni Mudra**

Yoni in Sanskriti means 'womb' or 'source' and is implicitly connected to the primary womb energy or the source of creation where senses are completely shut from the outer world. The final position of the fingers forms the womb shape.

Starting Position: Bring together the hands, touch the pads of the same fingers by keeping them straight and away from the body.

Variation 1:

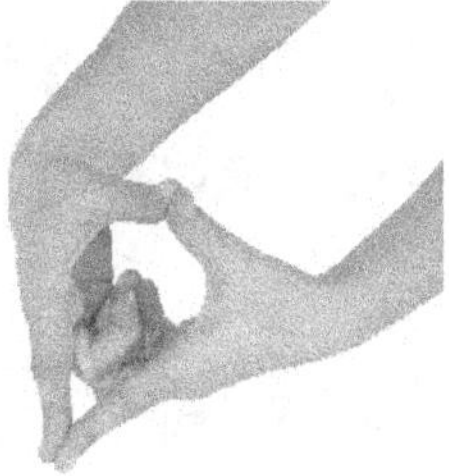

Turn the little, ring and middle finger inwards to interlock, so the backs of the fingers are touching. The thumbs' pads together should be looking towards the body and the index fingers; pads together should be pointed downwards.

Variation 2:

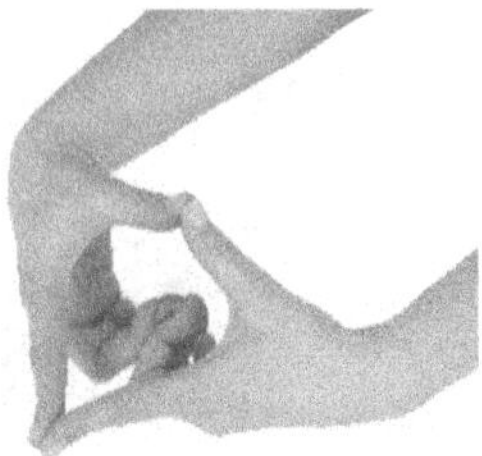

Can turn inward the little, ring and middle fingers, in which position, the front sides of the fingers should be touching. Each finger should be in contact with the same opposite hand finger.

Variation 3:

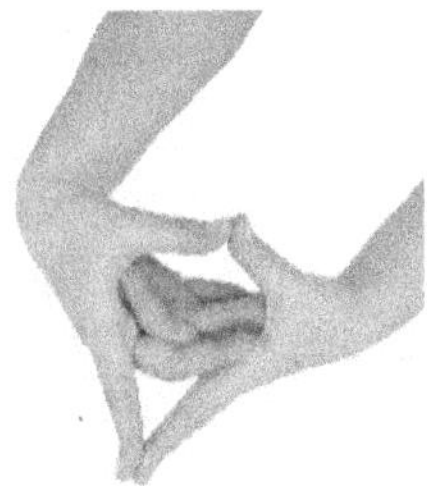

Can interlock the fingers lying open and flat on the inner palms, with the thumbs.

5.   **Fierce or Terrifying Attitude – Bhairava Mudra**

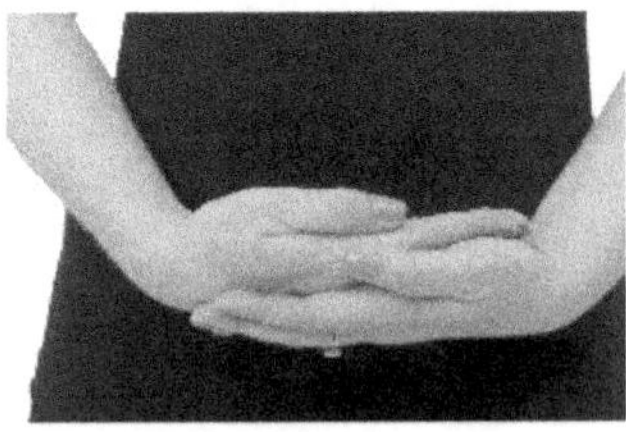

Place the right hand on top of the left with both palms facing upwards. Both hands should rest on the lap. The eyes should be closed and the body must be relaxed.

Note: When the left hand is on top, it is called Bhairavi Mudra which is corresponding to the female of Bhairava. The two hands represent the ida and pingala nadi and the connection of the practitioner with the divine and supreme consciousness.

6.   **Closing the Seven Gates – Shanmukhi Mudra**

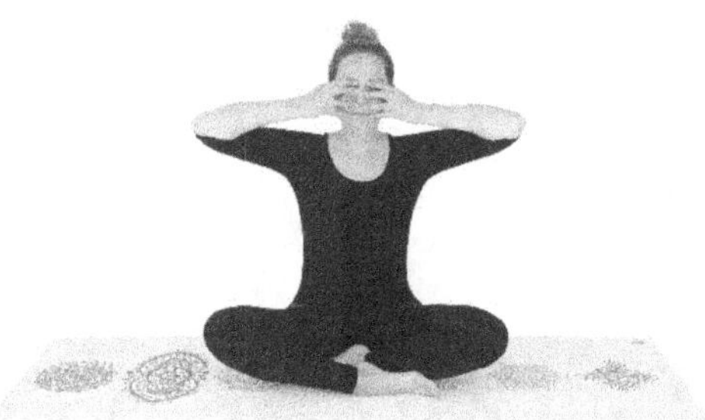

Raise the elbows and keep them parallel to the ground – this sitting position helps on focusing on the breathing. Close the eyes using the thumbs; the index fingers are gently placed on the eyelashes; the middle fingers are placed on top of the nostrils; the ring fingers are placed just below the nostrils and above the lips; the little fingers are placed at the brow of the lips.

Importance of Chanting

While yoga is not a religion, one could say that Om Chanting is. It is commonly used before prayers and during meditation in Hinduism, Buddhism and Jainism. However, with all the respect to the religious practicing, chanting can become a wonderful technique to travel within yourself and enhance focus, relaxation, activate chakras and balance your systems.

Keeping chakras activated, energy is rotated to its connected organ and glands which secrete hormones to influence and guide our emotional and physical being. There are many chakras that support the flow of prana or else life energy, however, the main chakras are seven and every one chants with a different sound, called Bija Mantra. Healing all chakras is important, in pregnancy though, most related is the sacral – swadhisthana chakra which helps strengthening the womb and balancing the secreted hormones for a smooth pregnancy. The vibrations from bija mantras chanting, naturally calm the nervous system, can create a sonic message for the baby and during labor and childbirth can help with the pain.

Chakra		Bija Mantra	Element	Energy	Action
Muladhara	Root	Lam	Earth	Safe, grounded	I am
Svadisthana	Sacral	Vam	Water	In the flow	I feel
Manipura	Solar plexus	Ram	Fire	Self-mastery	I do
Anahata	Heart	Yam	Air	Love	I love
Vishuddha	Throat	Ham	Ether	Creativity, expression, purification	I speak
Ajna	Third eye	Om or Aum	Light	Mind, wisdom	I see
Sahasrara	Crown	No chanting, focus on own self	The Supreme	Completeness, enlightenment	I know

By week 22, baby's hearing has developed and when the woman is exposed to chanting during her pregnancy, post birth the baby will have a familiar association with the sounds. During labor it can be helpful to ride the waves of contractions and use the bija mantras to release tension so with mental and physical awareness can cue the body to soften and open up for delivery.

Each bija mantra can be chanted out loud, known as Baikhari; whispering, known as Upanshu; or mentally, known as Manasik, which is the strongest and most difficult to practice as it is easy to lose concentration. It is not necessary to understand the meaning of the mantra, not the way of chanting, as long as there is awareness on the vibrations created and focus on the chakra area.

"Om" or "Aum" chanting is the most common one, and is characterized as the sound of the universe. When chanting "Om", the vibration resides in the throat, nose, sinuses, chest and heart space, which make it a powerful sound with a strong vibration. Chanting this bija mantra during pregnancy connects the mother to the creation of baby and life, and also can help on her empowerment as a woman. Other than strengthening the vocal cords and surrounding muscles when chanting, is helpful to open up the sinuses and reduce tension in the throat area, as well as reducing stress levels. It quiets the mind from any thoughts and enhances connection to self and universe.

Index of Asanas English – Sanskriti

S

T

Index of Asanas Sanskriti – English

Bibliography

1. Kerr MG, Scott DB & Samuel E (1964). *Studies of the inferior vena cava in late pregnancy.* BMJ 1, 532–533 – https://www.ncbi.nlm.nih.gov/pmc/articles/PMC1813561/

2. Swami Niranjanananda Saraswati (2016). *Prana and Pranayama.* New Delhi: Thomson Press (India) Limited

3. Swami Satyananda Saraswati (2012). *Yoga Nidra.* New Delhi: Thomson Press (India) Limited

4. From the Teachings of Swami Satyananda Saraswati Swami Niranjanananda Saraswati (2013). *Mudra Vigyan.* New Delhi: Thomson Press (India) Limited

5. Kumar P, Magon N. (2012) Hormones in pregnancy. Niger Med J. 53(4):179-183. Available from: https://www.ncbi.nlm.nih.gov/pubmed/23661874 [Accessed 11th July 2018]

6. MedlinePlus. (2016) Hormones. Available from: https://medlineplus.gov/hormones.html [Accessed 11th July 2018]

7. NHS Choices. (2018) Back pain in pregnancy. Available from: https://www.nhs.uk/conditions/pregnancy-and-baby/backache-pregnant/ [Accessed 11th July 2018]

8.   NHS Inform. (2017) Exercises during pregnancy. Available from: https://www.nhsinform.scot/healthy-living/keeping-active/getting-started/exercise-during-pregnancy [Accessed 11th July 2018]

9.   Northamptonshire Healthcare NHS Foundation Trust. (2015) Emotional changes during pregnancy and following childbirth. Available from: https://www.nhft.nhs.uk/download.cfm?doc=docm93jijm4n1351.pdf&ver=2068 [Accessed 11th July 2018]

10. Society for Endocrinology. (2018) You and your hormones. Hormones of pregnancy and labour. Available from: http://www.yourhormones.info/topical-issues/hormones-of-pregnancy-and-labour/ [Accessed 11th July 2018])